Health Risk Assessment: A Case-Based Approach

Health Risk Assessment: A Case-Based Approach

Edited by **Felix Rohmer**

New Jersey

Published by Foster Academics,
61 Van Reypen Street,
Jersey City, NJ 07306, USA
www.fosteracademics.com

Health Risk Assessment: A Case-Based Approach
Edited by Felix Rohmer

International Standard Book Number: 978-1-63242-224-8 (Hardback)

The publisher's policy is to use permanent paper from mills that operate a sustainable forestry policy. Furthermore, the publisher ensures that the text paper and cover boards used have met acceptable environmental accreditation standards.

Trademark Notice: Registered trademark of products or corporate names are used only for explanation and identification without intent to infringe.

Printed in the United States of America.

Contents

Permissions

List of Contributors

Preface

A descriptive account based on the field of health risk assessment has been presented in this elaborative book. It consists of a compilation of various health risk assessments for existing and rising hazards spanning a continuum. Psychoactive drug usage in drivers of delivery trucks and using look-back risk evaluation for accidental syringe re-use in healthcare settings are some of the case studies on existing risks covered in this book. Case studies regarding rising risks include precautionary actions to protect blood supplies; deposition of nanoparticles in the lung; and the epistemic issues related to genetically enhanced organism risk evaluations. The book also highlights progressing health risk assessment analysis through a post-genomics lens and elucidates the case studies on personalized genomics, advancing in silico models for risk evaluation and novel data analyses.

The information contained in this book is the result of intensive hard work done by researchers in this field. All due efforts have been made to make this book serve as a complete guiding source for students and researchers. The topics in this book have been comprehensively explained to help readers understand the growing trends in the field.

I would like to thank the entire group of writers who made sincere efforts in this book and my family who supported me in my efforts of working on this book. I take this opportunity to thank all those who have been a guiding force throughout my life.

Editor

Part 1

Typical Health Risk Assessment Case Studies for Novel Risks

Professional Drivers and Psychoactive Substances Consumption: First Results from Medical Surveillance at the Workplace in Italy

Gian Luca Rosso[1,*], Mauro Feola[2], Maria Paola Rubinetto[3],
Nicola Petti[3] and Lorenzo Rubinetto[3]
[1]Occupational Health Physician
Occupational Health Physician, S.C. Emergenza Urgenza 118, Cuneo,
[2]Riabilitazione Cardiologica – Unità Scompenso Cardiaco,
Ospedale SS Trinità Fossano (CN),
[3]Se.M. s.r.l. Medical Services, Cuneo,
Italy

1. Introduction

The role played by psychoactive substances in work safety has recently become the object of increasing interest in Italy [1,2]. Particularly for professional drivers, these substances can reduce driving performance and increase the risk of accidents with fatal outcomes not only for workers but also for third parties [3]. Even if the accountability of psychotropic drugs as a cause of work accidents remains difficult to evaluate with precision, there is much evidence that the use of psychoactive substances is a major risk factor for accidents by professional drivers [4,5].

Until 2008, it was not permitted to investigate the use of psychoactive substances among any worker's category in Italy. After promulgation of two recent Italian laws (the first published in the Official Gazette No. 266, November 15, 2007, and the second came into force in May 2008, the Legislative Decree 81/08), the occupational health physician (the so-called "Competent Physician") is called to assess the use of illicit drugs among professional drivers, in order to detect dependency at the workplace and improve the security and health of workers and others [6].

This Legislative Decree (DL 81/08) seemed to reiterate the importance of exceeding the simple concept of health protection of the worker, as conceived by the Legislative Decree 626/94, to reach a more comprehensive analysis of all complex work activities and all special risks to security and the health of others.

A recent Study Group on Hazardous Workers, conducted in Italy (La.R.A. Group) [3], has estimated between 4% to 10% of Italian workers may be drugs consumers. There are no previous studies that have analysed this phenomenon (by testing the illegal substances or

---

* Corresponding Author

their metabolite in blood or urine) in Italian professional drivers or in any other worker category.

The main purpose of this study was to investigate the prevalence of psychoactive substance usage among professional drivers by rapid urine analysis for the majority of often used illicit drugs.

2. Materials and methods

The study group included 198 professional drivers from 47 companies in Piedmont Region. From July to December 2008 each worker was investigated with a rapid urine screening test. In case of positive testing results the physician responsible for medical surveillance of workers defines the employee as "temporarily unfit". In order to verify this finding, the positive urine samples were sent to a specialized laboratory to confirm the previous results. Workers positive for drug tests were referred to a public health institution for diagnostic classification (drugs use, abuse or dependence) and treatment.

2.1 Companies and categories of professional drivers involved

Forty-seven companies (with at least one work site in Piedmont Region) were involved in the study. All of these companies have one or more workers employed as professional drivers. In our experience we have defined professional drivers as the workers involved in driving trucks or other vehicles (forklift trucks, dollies, excavators, diggers etc.). We have considered all tasks that required the driver to stay at the wheel (for more than a half working hour) with a very good reaction capacity and a high level of attention. Professional drivers were divided into three groups:

1. truckers: 69 subjects, 9/69 were personal chauffeurs (only class B license required), the other 60/69 were truck drivers;
2. warehousemen: 104 workers involved in driving forklift trucks or dollies in workshop and/or depots;
3. construction workers: 25 drivers of heavy vehicles used for excavation (excavators or diggers) working in building yards.

The main features of the study population are indicated in table 1.

2.2 Rapid urine screening tests

According to the recent indications of the major Italian studies, we tested workers' urine for illicit substances or their metabolites using a rapid urine screening test. For the rapid urine screening test we used a multi-drug, one step, multi-line screen test device (SureStep Multi-Drug, Innovacon, Inc. Manufacturer), an immunoassay test based on the principle of competitive binding. A drug, if present in the urine, reacts with its specific antibody and a visible colored line will show up in the test line region of the specific drug strip. This test was used only for the qualitative detection of the following psychoactive substances (the cut-off level is expressed in ng/mL): amphetamines (AMP, 500), barbiturates (BARB, 300), benzodiazepines (BZO, 300), tetrahydrocannabinol (THC, 50), methadone (MTD, 300), opiates (OPI, 300), cocaine (COC, 300), MethyleneDioxyMethaAmphetamine (MDMA, 500), phencyclidine (PCP, 25), and tricyclic antidepressants (TCA, 1000).

Professional Drivers and Psychoactive Substances Consumption: First Results from Medical Surveillance at the Workplace in Italy

5

2.3 Clinical research protocol

Upon admission, each subject was informed of the provisions related to the medical surveillance of drug dependency at the workplace. At least one month before the screening test, it was explained to each worker that the occupational health physician would have to investigate the use of illicit drugs among professional drivers. It was also explained that the identification of positive rapid urine screening test would cause a temporarily unfit judgment to any complex working activities (such as professional driving) and may also cause a temporary loss of job.

For the achievement of these aims we have adopted the following procedural algorithm (figure 1):

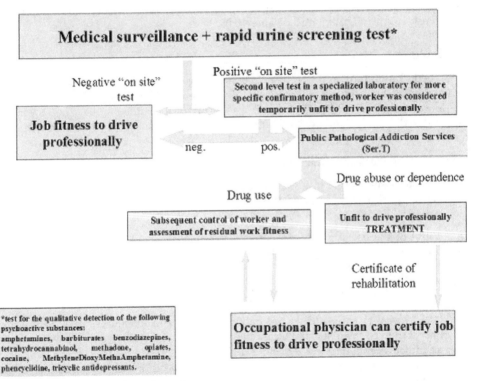

Fig. 1. Procedural algorithm adopted

- *Communication stage*: the initial phase, in which each worker was informed that the identification of positive rapid urine screening test would cause a temporarily unfit judgment to any complex working activities (such as professional drive) and may also cause a temporary loss of job.
- *Samples collection stage for first level tests:* professional drivers were convened with a written notice only 1 day before the analysis (in order to avoid intentional suspensions of drugs assumption). During medical surveillance of workers the occupational physician analyzed urine samples from employees with the rapid screening test.

- *Stage of urine sample preservation for second level tests*: only in the case of a positive screening test would the physician seal the urine sample (in the presence of the worker) and send it to a specialized laboratory to obtain a confirmed result.
- "Job fitness" stage: workers positive for drug tests were considered temporarily unfit to drive professionally and referred to a public Pathological Addiction Services (Ser.T.) for diagnostic classification (drugs use, abuse or dependence) and treatment.

2.4 Statistical analysis

Continuous variables are summarized by the mean (M) and the standard deviation (S.D.). Two independent samples t-test (unpaired) was used to compare differences between variables in professional drivers with positive or negative test. Categorical variables were analyzed using the chi-square test. All probability values were two-tailed and differences were considered significant with a p value ≤ 0.05.

3. Results

In the period from July until December 2008 rapid urine screening test was carried out on 198 workers. All subjects were professional drivers (employees who spend more than half the time at the wheel): 69 (34.8%) truck drivers or personal chauffeurs, 104 (52.6%) workers involved in drive machinery for the handling of goods (lift truck), and 25 (12.6%) drivers of machinery for the moving of earth.

Main results and features of the study population are indicated in table 1.

We found 14 positive rapid urine screening test (7.1%) and these results from the screening stage were verified by specialized laboratories. The results of the second level tests are indicated in table 2.

One (7.1%) of the positive test was not confirmed and one (7.1%) was positive only for benzodiazepines. Considering only illegal substances were detected, 6.1% of all drivers tested positive (12/198 professional drivers). Cannabis (THC) was the most frequently detected substance (seen in 83.3% of cases), after that was the methadone (16.7%) and then cocaine (8.3%). In only one subject more than one substance was found (THC and COC).

Five (41.7%) were ex drug-addicts and public Pathological Addiction Services (Ser.T.) had previously followed them. It is important to emphasize that these workers had not declared their ex addiction until they tested positive at the screening test. As for the other 7 (58.3%), it was the first time they tested positive and, on the basis of history and clinical examination, an addiction was excluded. Despite those considerations, all 12 positive workers underwent assessment at Ser.T (as indicated by Italian laws) for diagnostic classification (drugs use, abuse or dependence, but on the basis of illicit drugs values, 2% of professional drivers investigated were assumed to be drug abusers) and treatment.

We have not found significant differences in illicit drug consumption between the three groups analyzed. A trend in favour of attitude to drug assumption among workers involved in drive machinery for the handling of goods emerged.

In our study professional drivers from 31 to 35 years old have a higher risk to be consumers than younger drivers (p=.015), as shown in table 3. However, it should be noted that the

Professional Drivers and Psychoactive Substances Consumption: First Results from Medical Surveillance at the Workplace in Italy

7

		Truck drivers or personal chauffeurs	Drivers of machinery for the handling of goods	Drivers of machinery for the moving of earth
Age [years; M (S.D.)]		41 (10.1)	40 (8.6)	40 (12.8)
Distribution by age groups	18 - 30 years	13	24	7
	31 - 40 years	15	41	7
	41 - 50 years	28	30	6
	51 - 71 years	13	9	5
Total		69	104	25
Sex		68 M 1F	101 M 3F	25 M 0F
Mean duration of employment [years; M (S.D.)]		13 (10.5)	11 (6.7)	14 (14)
Educational level [n (%)]	Elementary	3 (4.4%)	1 (0.9%)	1 (4%)
	Middle school	53 (76.8%)	65 (62.5%)	15 (60%)
	High school	13 (18.8%)	37 (35.7%)	9 (36%)
	University	-	1 (0.9%)	-
Positivity "on site" tests, confirmed at second level tests [n (%)]	THC	2 (2.9%)	8 (7.7%)	-
	COC	1 (1.4%)	-	-
	MTD	1 (1.4%)	1 (1%)	-
	BZO	1 (1.4%)	-	-

M= Mean and S.D.=standard deviation

Table 1. Main features of the study population for three professional driver categories for age distribution, sex, emplyment duration, education level and positivity

Test	Positive [n (%)]	Concentrations [ng/ml (S.D.)]	Cut-off (ng/mL)
Tetrahydrocannabinol (THC)	10 (5.1%)	62.2 (64)	15
Cocaine (COC)	1 (0.5%)	4603	100
Benzodiazepines (BZO)	1 (0.5%)	-	-
Methadone (MTD)	2 (1%)	2542 (984.3)	100

Table 2. Drug types and values for the professional drivers that tested positive.

mean age of the study population was around 40 years old and the largest group was between 31 and 50 years old. The distribution of positive tests by age groups is as follows:

- under 31 years: 44 subjects, none tested positive,
- age between 31 and 40 years: 8 out of 63 positive for THC, COC and MTD,
- age between 41 and 50 years: 64 workers, two positive to THC,
- over fifty years: 27 subjects, two positive to THC and MTD.

In our sample the mean age of THC consumers is 38.3 (S.D. 6.93), this result is apparently in contrast with data from international literature, in particular a French study showed that THC use by truck drivers was higher in younger workers (age between 18 and 25 years) [7]. With the exception of one subject (THC positive with a value of 238 ng/ml), the other nine were feebly positive to THC, in fact all THC urine values were beneath the 80 ng/ml.

One female worker proved to be positive to THC, despite the small number of women enrolled.

We have not found significant differences in the mean duration of employment or educational level between workers that tested positive. However, in our sample, workers who were positive seemed to have a mean duration of employment lower than the negative ones (see table 3).

AGE	NEGATIVE	POSITIVE	P
≤ 30 years	44	0	0.015*
31 – 35 years	29	6	
31 – 35 years	29	6	0.122
≥ 36 years	113	6	
≤ 30 years	44	0	0.29
≥ 36 years	113	6	
DURATION OF EMPLOYMENT [years; M (S.D.)]	11.3 (9.6)	8.1 (6.7)	0.15
MEAN AGE [years; M (S.D.)]	39.1 (9.9)	39 (7.6)	0.9

* significant

Table 3. Age and duration of employment of the study subjects

For the professional driver who was found positive to BZN, we have not adopted the procedural algorithm in figure 1, but we have decided to intensify the medical surveillance of the workers. None of 198 subjects tested positive to TCA or BARB.

The 12 workers identified positive to the rapid urine screening test, were judged to be temporarily unfit to drive professionally and, three of those (25%) suffered a temporary loss of their job, the other nine were placed in other working activities. This consequence is related to the small size of the companies within the study (such as many of Italian transportation companies) which had great difficulties placing their professional drivers in another working activity [6].

Finally, positive cases were dispersed between the 47 companies, without bias towards any one driving group that may suggest a critical situation in one or more companies.

4. Discussion

The most significant result in this study is the prevalence of employees (more than 6%, between those involved in complex working activities) that, with different modalities, have a problem of substances consumption. Nevertheless, the analysis of the current findings requires cautions: in fact, if we exclude the workers who tested positive for THC only (in

Professional Drivers and Psychoactive Substances Consumption: First Results from Medical Surveillance at the Workplace in Italy

9

low concentrations) or BZN, we would be left with a small group of four professional drivers (2%) who tested positive to COC or MTD or THC (in high concentrations). These four workers are particularly dangerous for themselves and also for third parties. On the other hand, we should not underestimate the current results because, despite all 198 workers being informed beforehand of the provisions related to screening test, 12 employees were not able to stop their consumption of illicit drugs.

Cannabis was the most frequently detected substance (seen in 83.3% of positive cases). This observation matches the previous studies conducted in other countries, which have indicated cannabis as the principal illicit drug consumed by drivers [8,9]. Moreover, the distribution of illicit drugs among professional drivers is similar to a previous published French experience [7].

The major limitation of this study is the small population examined, which may limit generalization of the findings.

In our study, the risk for consumption of illicit drugs between professional drivers aged 31 and 40 years old seemed to be higher. This result may be due to the fact that younger workers are probably concerned about losing their job (they usually have atypical employment contracts or they work without contracts). However these results confirm that in Italy, the problem concerning substance consumptions in complex working activities is not restricted to a certain age of workers but actually involves all age groups. It should be noted that our sample was relatively small; therefore we did not find significant differences in mean duration of employment and/or educational level between workers who tested positive and negative ones.

The rapid urine screening test, which we have used in our study, was a useful tool. The two cases, in which the test "on site" was not confirmed by specialized laboratory, are probably due to the lack of physician experience which may have caused the erroneous reading. It is also important to point out that a positive result does not indicate intoxication and does not mean that behavioral abilities are impaired during working activity. It should be recalled that there is no clear association between occasional use of psychoactive substances like THC and increased risk for work accidents; however, cannabis use can amplify the other risk factors associated with accidents and injuries [10].

In the current study, 25% of worker who tested positive have suffered a temporary loss of their job, but none of those was defined with certainty as a drug abuser. This situation is due to the fact that the 47 companies in the study are small in size (as are many of the Italian transportation companies) and they have difficulties placing a professional driver in another working activity [11]. Furthermore, at the end of this study only one out of 12 professional drivers was evaluated by Ser.T, because the time it takes to call him in requires several weeks.

To our knowledge, this is the first Italian research study that has investigated the use of psychoactive substances among professional drivers using urine analysis to detect many of the major illicit drugs. Our results highlight that the problem of drug consumption among professional drivers in Italy is real. Health education (with new prevention programmes able to involve all age groups) and medical surveillance (with workplace drug-testing) may improve the safety of workers and also third parties.

5. Acknowledgment

This study was totally self supporting. Part of the results of this article has been presented at the national congress of SIMLII held in Turin in 2011.

We thank the technicians and physician of the S. Luigi Hospital Orbassano (TO) for the collaboration and help confirming the rapid urine tests.

6. References

[1] M.M. Ferrario, P. Apostoli, P.A. Bertazzi, G. Cesana, G. Mosconi, L. Riboldi, Occupational medicine faces new health challenges: the example of alcohol dependence, Med. Lav. 98 (2007) 355-373.

[2] F. Spigno, N. Debarbieri, F. Traversa, Workplace and psychoactive substances dependence: certificate of eligibility for work and perspectives of prevention in the light of recent innovative regulations, G. Ital. Med. Lav. Erg. 29 (2007) 158-165.

[3] N. Magnavita, A. Bergamaschi, M. Chiarotti, A. Colombi, B. Deidda, G. De lorenzo, Workers with alcohol and drug addiction problems Consensus Document of the Study Group on Hazardous Workers, Med. Lav. 99 (2008) 3-58.

[4] I.M. Bernhoft, A. Steentoft, S.S. Johansen, N.A. Klitgaard, L.B. Larsen, L.B. Hansen, Drugs in injured drivers in Denmark, Forensic Sci. Int. 150 (2005) 181-189.

[5] J.G. Bramness, S. Skurtveit, J. Morland, Clinical impairment of benzodiazepines-relation between benzodiazepine concentrations and impairment in apprehended drivers, Drug Alcohol Depend. 68 (2002) 131-141.

[6] G.L. Rosso, R. Zanelli, S. Bruno, M. Feola, M. Bobbio, Professional driving and safety, a target for occupational medicine, Med. Lav. 98 (2007) 355-373.

[7] L. Labat, B. Fontaine, C. Delzenne, A. Doublet, M.C. Marek, D. Tellier, M. Tonneau, M. Lhermitte, P. Frimat, Prevalence of psychoactive substances in truck drivers in the Nord-Pas-de-Calais region (France), Forensic Sci. Int. 174 (2008) 90-94.

[8] B.M. Appenzeller, S. Schneider, M. Yegles, A. Maul, R. Wennig, Drugs and chronic alcohol abuse in drivers, Forensic Sci. Int. 155 (2005) 83-90.

[9] O.H. Drummer, J. Gerostamoulos, H. Batziris, M. Chu, J.R. Caplehorn, M.D. Robertson, P. Swann, The incidence of drugs in drivers killed in Australian road traffic crashes, Forensic Sci. Int. 134 (2003) 154-162.

[10] E.J. Wadsworth, S.C. Moss, S.A. Simpson, A.P. Smith, A community based investigation of the association between cannabis use, injuries and accidents, J. Psychopharmacol. 20 (2006) 5-13.

[11] G.L. Rosso, Prevention of road accidents involving heavy vehicles, what role for occupational medicine?, G. Ital. Med. Lav. Ergon. 30 (2008) 309-311.

2

The Risk of Blood-Borne Viral Infection due to Syringe Re-Use

Tamer Oraby et al.*
McLaughlin Centre for Population Health Risk Assessment, University of Ottawa,
Canada

1. Introduction

Transmission of viral and bacterial infections through the practice of syringe re-use has been repeatedly documented (American Society of Anesthesiologists, 1999) and controlled experiments have demonstrated that a syringe barrel becomes contaminated with microbes after multiple re-uses (Lessard et al., 1988; Perceval, 1980).

In the fall of 2008, light was shed on the practice of syringe re-use occurring in western Canada (Government of Alberta, 2009). In this situation, syringes had been re-used between patients to administer sedating medication through patient intravenous (IV) lines (Government of Alberta, 2009). Later it was reported that other incidents of syringe re-use had occurred in Canada (CBC News-Edmonton, 2008a;CBC News-Edmonton, 2008b). The question arose of whether this practice may have resulted in the transmission of blood-borne pathogens to patients and, if so, how many and with what level of risk. To answer this question, a retrospective study involving approximately 1,400 patients was undertaken (Government of Alberta, 2009). However, questions were also raised as to whether estimates based on modeling scenarios could provide information to guide decisions on the need for look-backs.

Risk assessments have been carried out almost concurrently with the underlying study; they gave various and different conclusions (Population Health Branch-Saskatchewan Health, 2009; Sikora et al., 2010). Contrary to our study where we considered the Canadian nation as a whole, the Population Health Branch-Saskatchewan study looked at only a province-wide risk assessment for Saskatchewan based on the same methods in Sikora et al. (2010); they concluded that the blood-borne viral infection was negligible (Population Health Branch-

* Susie Elsaadany[2,**], Robert Gervais[2], Mustafa Al-Zoughool[1], Michael G. Tyshenko[1], Lynn Johnston[3], Mel Krajden[4], Dick Zoutman[5], Jun Wu[2] and Daniel Krewski[1,6]
[1]*McLaughlin Center for Population Health Risk Assessment, University of Ottawa, Ottawa, Canada,*
[2]*Public Health Agency of Canada, Ottawa, Canada,*
[3]*Queen Elizabeth II Health Sciences Centre, Nova Scotia, Canada,*
[4]*BC Centre for Disease Control, University of British Columbia, Vancouver, Canada,*
[5]*Medical Microbiology and Infection Control, Queen's University, Ontario, Canada,*
[6]*Department of Epidemiology and Community Medicine, Faculty of Medicine, University of Ottawa, Ottawa, Canada*
** Corresponding Author

Saskatchewan Health, 2009). The model in Sikora et al., (2010) is a multiplicative model of four probabilities. It also considers only the risk that one patient is imposing on one other patient without taking into account the number of times the syringe may have been re-used in between them.

A novel but simple probabilistic model is established in the underlying study to reflect more accurately the practical situation that is occurring. The risk of viral infection at any time of re-use depends not only on the prevalence and susceptibility but also the number of times the syringe barrel was re-used before that time. Uncertainty and sensitivity analyses were carried out here to incorporate the lack of knowledge about different parameters, e.g. probability of contaminating a syringe, and assess their influence on the risk.

2. Methods

Blood-borne diseases can be transmitted through contact with bodily fluids, most often blood; they include Hepatitis B (HBV), Hepatitis C (HCV) and Human Immunodeficiency Virus (HIV). A probabilistic model was designed for the purpose of assessing the risk of these three viral infections due to re-use of syringes on multiple patients. The values for multiple risk factor variables used in this quantitative risk assessment were obtained from the literature (where data existed), consensus of opinions from a nationally commissioned expert working group, (Public Health Agency of Canada, 2008; Public Health Agency of Canada, 2009) and from information extracted from recently documented cases of syringe re-use in Canada and other countries.

The risk assessment consisted of three main areas: 1) Issue identification, 2) Exposure and hazard assessment, and 3) Hazard and risk characterization.

2.1 Issue identification

There are many different types of IV apparatus systems, with possibly thousands of combinations of add-on auxiliary components. This assessment investigated the constituents of a basic IV administration apparatus, and the components of a generic disposable plastic syringe to choose a "most common method" used by health care workers to deliver medications to patients via the intravenous route. The apparatus chosen is described in the exposure and hazard assessment section below.

2.2 Exposure and hazard assessment

To provide preliminary estimates of the level of exposure to viral pathogens via plastic syringe re-use, assumptions in the following categories were defined:

a.   Assumptions of health care worker (HCW) practices

The precise number of times an HCW will re-use a syringe is unknown, and independent of the number of times the syringe was re-used previously.

b.   Assumptions about medical device/instrument properties

Contamination of the syringe/tubing via fluid backflow was estimated based on the proximity of the medication injection site to the patient. A generic instrument set up was used, which consisted of an infusion bag, and a length of tubing long enough to have a significant fluid flow/possibility of wash-out between two sites of injection; one proximal injection site at the bag, one distal at the catheter. No filters, locks or check valves were taken into account.

c.   Assumptions on patient characteristics and needs

Patients treated are randomly selected from a high risk population on which the syringe could have been re-used; virus carriers can potentially infect any of the subsequent patients in a group before a syringe is disposed; and the events of source patient infection, virus contamination of the syringe and transmitting virus to subsequent patients are independent.

d.   Assumptions on the nature of the viruses targeted

In accordance with worst case scenario, the presence of virus in the blood of a model patient is binary (either yes or no); the infectivity of the virus is 100%.

This assessment addresses only potential infection with re-used syringes. Other potential sources of contamination, in particular the contamination of multi-dose medicine vials, are not considered due to the lack of sufficient information in the literature.

2.3 Hazard and risk characterization

The model used probabilistic designed to assess the risk of HIV, HCV and HBV infection attributed to syringe re-use on multiple patients. The risk of viral contamination and subsequent patient infection only arises if the syringe is re-used. It is also changing with the number of syringe re-uses (S), or equivalently with the number of previous infectious patients on whom the syringe was re-used ($R_1, R_2, R_3, ...$). The risk is lowered, but not completely eliminated, by a log reduction factor, if the syringe is flushed (this is known as "wash-out").

If s patients were known to have been exposed to a re-used syringe, the risk of viral infection for the kth patient in the sequence of s patients could be determined. The risk that the patient number k will contract the viral infection from one of the previous $k - 1$ patients is given by:

$$R_k = P^{(sus)} \times \left[1 - \prod_{j=1}^{k-1} \left(1 - Prev \times P^{(cont)} \times P_{k-j}^{(trans)} \right) \right], \text{for } k = 2, ..., s \qquad (1)$$

with $R_1 = 0$, where $Prev$ is the prevalence, $P^{(cont)}$ is the probability of contaminating the syringe, $P^{(cont)}$ is the probability of being susceptible and $P_{k-j}^{(trans)}$ is the probability of transmitting the disease after $k - j - 1$ usages. The individual risk ($Risk$), or the risk imposed on a patient that underwent syringe re-use practice, is given by:

$$Risk = P(practice) \times \sum_{s=2}^{\infty} \frac{1}{s} \sum_{k=1}^{s} R_k \times P(S = s) \qquad (2)$$

Here, S can be denoted as the number of injections until syringe replacement. The random variable S follows a geometric distribution with mean number of re-uses M given that $S \geq 2$. Thus, the individual risk is given by:

$$Risk = P(practice) \times \frac{1}{M-1} \times \sum_{s=2}^{\infty} \frac{1}{s} \sum_{k=1}^{s} R_k \times \left(1 - \frac{1}{M-1}\right)^{s-2} \tag{3}$$

where $P(practice)$ is the probability of syringe re-use practice. While the derivation of the three equations is straightforward, proofs are given in Appendix 1 for completion. Table 1 describes the model components and the values used to run the analysis.

Component	Variable	Range or Description	Probability Distribution*
Syringe re-use practice	$P(practice)$	2.2% - 60%	Pert (2.2%, 20%, 60%)
Wash-out factor	$r = 10^v$	Log-reduction	Uniform (1,2)
HBV immunity	Pro_{immu}	47%[1]	Triangular (46%, 47%, 48%)
HBV immunized but infected	$Pro_{immu\ and\ infected}$	4%†	Triangular (3.5%, 4%, 4.5%)
# of patients in one group	S	Geometrically distributed	Discrete Triangular (2, 6,10)
Mean # of patients in one group	M	2-10	
Prevalence HIV HCV HBV	$Prev$	0.1% - 1.5% 2% - 4% 0.5% - 4%	Pert (0.1%, 0.4%, 1.5%) Pert (0.5%, 2%, 4%) Pert (0.5%, 1%, 3%)
Transmission HIV HCV HBV	$P_d^{(trans)}$	(0.3% - 0.5%) × (wash-out factor)[2] (1% - 3%) × (wash-out factor) (10% - 30%) × (wash-out factor)	Triangular (0.3%, 0.4%, 0.5%) Triangular (1%, 2%, 3%) Triangular (10%, 20%, 30%)
Susceptibility HIV HCV HBV	$p^{(sus)}$	$1 - Prev$ $1 - Prev$ $1 - (Prev + Pro_{immu} - Pro_{immu\ and\ infected})$	
Contamination Proximal Distal	$p^{(cont)}$	3.3% 0.3%	Triangular (2.3%, 3.3%, 4.3%) Triangular (0.2%, 0.3%, 0.4%)

* Pert (min, most likely, max), Triangular (min, most likely, max) and Uniform (min, max)

Table 1. Model components with the values and distributions used for the MCS analysis

Monte Carlo Simulations (MCS) were necessary to incorporate uncertainties surrounding syringe re-use practice. MCS sometimes requires specific computational software and platforms. In this study, we have used Monte Carlo Simulations implemented on the R statistical software (R Development Core Team, 2010).

---

[1] Refer to Table 2.

[2] The efficiency of transmission is calculated by multiplying transmission percentage by log reduction (wash-out) factors.

The parameter "Pro_{immu}" represents the percentage of individuals who display HBV immunity after having received HBV vaccination. The immunogenicity of the HBV vaccine is not 100%, and requires multiple dosing to achieve protective antibody levels (≥ 10 IU/L) (Mackie et al., 2009). The primary determinant of seroprotection is the age at which an individual is vaccinated. The average HBV seroprotection rates as described by the Canadian Immunization Guide (Public Health Agency of Canada, 2006) are outlined in Table 2.

Age Range (years)	Seroprotection Rates
>2	95%
5-15	99%
20-29	95%
30-39	90%
40-49	86%
50-59	71%
≥ 60	50% to 70%

Table 2. Seroprotection rates based on age groups following HBV vaccination, data from The Canadian Immunization Guide (Public Health Agency of Canada, 2006)

Recipient factors other than age also affect the rate of seroprotection in vaccinated individuals. For example, the antibody response is lower in patients with diabetes mellitus (range: 70% to 80%), renal failure (range: 60% to 70%) and chronic liver disease (range: 60% to 70%). Based on these factors, as well as vaccination uptake in the population, the expert group working on this assessment concluded that approximately 47% (range: 46% to 48%) of the general population is susceptible to HBV infection due to the absence of protective levels of antibodies to HBV in the year 2008 (Mackie et al., 2009; Public Health Agency of Canada, 2006).

The parameter "$Pro_{immu\ and\ infected}$" represents the percentage of individuals who are HBV infected, and who have also been vaccinated against HBV, as of the year 2008. The value was determined through expert consensus of a nationally organized working group (Public Health Agency of Canada, 2008).

Finally, a set of input distributions needed to be created for each variable, in order to run the MCS analysis. Using information provided by health care experts (Public Health Agency of Canada, 2009), we arrived at a set of distributions to address the uncertainty involved in syringe re-use (Table 1).

3. Results

Scenario analysis was conducted for each blood-borne viral infection using different input values and distributions (Table 1). For the three blood-borne viral infections, the model was most sensitive to changes in disease prevalence. For example, changing the prevalence of HIV from 0.004 to 0.015 increased the individual risk by about 4 times (0.161 and 0.596, respectively) for a value of average syringe re-use of 4 and a wash-out factor of 100. Similarly for HBV, increasing the prevalence from 0.005 to 0.030 increased the individual risk from 6.911 to 43.60, when using an average value of syringe re-use of 4 and a wash-out factor of 100. The increase in risk is almost linear in the disease prevalence, which is supported by the sensitivity analysis (Appendix 2).

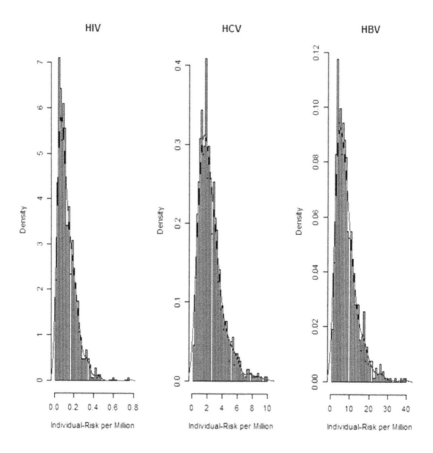

Fig. 1. Probability density function of individual risk of viral infection (y-axis) for HIV, HCV, and HBV per million person-procedures (x-axis) for the proximal setting scenario.

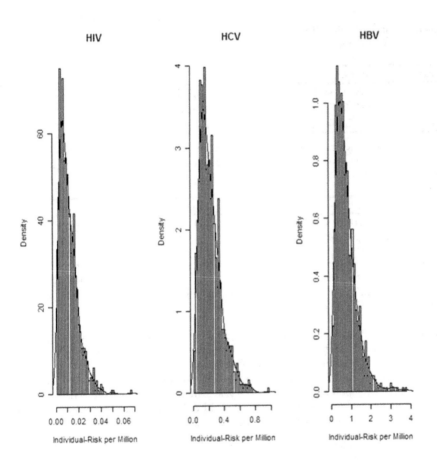

Fig. 2. Probability density function of individual risk of viral infection (y-axis) for HIV, HCV, and HBV per million person-procedures (x-axis) for the distal setting scenario.

Analysis of the resultant probability density functions (refer to Figures 1 and 2) of the individual risk per million person-procedure indicates that the distribution is right-skewed for the three infections for both proximal and distal injection into IV lines. The dispersion is relatively close in both settings for each viral infection. However, the median risk (used for skewness concerns) in the distal setting is about 10% of that resulted for the proximal setting similar to what was found in a study by Perceval (1980). This indicates that individual risk of viral contamination is highly dependent on whether injection takes place at a site proximal or distal to the IV set.

Table 3 and Table 4 present the individual risk per million people for proximal and distal medication injection sites. It is clear that the risk of HBV is highest in both settings due the higher efficacy of transmission inherent in the nature of the virus.

Virus	95% CI	Mean	Median	Coefficient of Variation
HIV	[0.0205, 0.3361]	0.1248927	0.1030704	0.6939076
HCV	[0.4584, 6.2700]	2.430697	2.090218	0.6436132
HBV	[1.7917, 21.8748]	8.292251	7.016490	0.6660043

Table 3. Output of the uncertainty analysis- the mean, median and coefficient of variation for the individual risk per million person procedure for a medication injection site that is *proximal* to the patient's IV set

Virus	95% CI	Mean	Median	Coefficient of Variation
HIV	[0.0017, 0.0313]	0.01138309	0.009550734	0.6966828
HCV	[0.0407,0.5597]	0.2197540	0.1911161	0.6202549
HBV	[0.1487, 2.0497]	0.7553183	0.6323613	0.6755055

Table 4. Output of the uncertainty analysis- the mean, median and coefficient of variation for the individual risk per million person procedure for a medication injection site that is *distal* to the patient's IV set

A Monte Carlo Bayesian sensitivity analysis was performed, using the "tgp" package (Gramacy & Taddy, 2009) on the R statistical software (R Development Core Team, 2010). From a series of box plots (attached in Appendix 2) it is clear that prevalence, especially of HIV and HBV, should be considered in future analyses to identify the risk of patient infection with viral pathogens following syringe re-use. In the case of HIV, resolving the uncertainty surrounding prevalence alone would reduce the total variance by 45%, while it takes all other factors combined to contribute the same magnitude of effect.

Additionally, it appears the main effect due to changes in the prevalence is linear (results not shown here but available upon request). The probability of (re-use) practice and the efficacies of transmission and contamination follow the prevalence in their influence and linear effect on the output. The remaining factors can be fixed to any value within their range without significantly impacting the output.

4. Discussion

The model estimated a broad range of infection risk for HIV, HCV, and HBV transmission through syringe re-use in the health care setting, as of the year 2008. The model estimated the risk of contracting infection after syringe re-use to range from .02 - .34 in a million person-procedure for HIV; from .5 - 6.3 in a million person-procedure for HCV; and from 1.8 - 21.8 in a million person-procedure for HBV. Moreover, vulnerable groups with reduced seroprotection and reduced immunity may experience more severe outcomes if exposed to blood-borne viruses by this route.

In a similar study it was concluded that the risk of HBV on the Canadian population is highest in the proximal setting with risk of infection 12 - 53 per million followed by HCV (1 - 4.3 per million) and HIV (.03 - .15 per million) (Sikora et al., 2010). The last two ranges are subsets of the ranges we give above while the probability of practice used in Sikora et al. (2010) is 20% - 80% which is higher than the range we used 2.2% - 60%. The risk of HBV is smaller in our results may be because the Population Health Branch-Saskatchewan Health study focused on the Albertan population when the authors estimated probability of susceptibility for HBV (Population Health Branch-Saskatchewan Health, 2009).

The worst-case scenario risk assessment detailed here focuses on this event of syringe re-use as a way to quantify levels of risk for blood-borne viruses, to provide risk assessment information for better decision making, and to identify public health risk management lessons. Calculations were performed using the best available data at the time of this incident; the data used here are for the years 2008-2009. The authors acknowledge the fact that more and better data have become and will continue to become available. This risk assessment model allows for adaptation, further refinements, and future re-assessments based on improved input data.

One of the more interesting and important outcomes of the modeling, is the identification of information gaps and sources of uncertainty in this kind of analysis. We identified a number of information gap areas that are amenable for improvement. First, there was substantial uncertainty surrounding the time period of events in this model. For example, the publication of guidelines in 1995 and 1996 must have had a time dependent effect on the practice of syringe re-use. Changes in syringe re-use practice over time were incorporated by using a wide range of probability, from a 2.2% chance of re-use to a 60% chance. As it is assumed that syringe re-use practice is decreasing, then the model may well have overestimated the probability of acquiring infection.

Second, substantial uncertainty exists around the nature of the viruses targeted in this model context. Several aspects of the dose-response relationship and infectivity of the three viruses have been treated in a simplified manner to account for uncertainty around the potential concentration of the HBV/HCV/HIV within one exposure unit, the volumetric quantity to be considered a single exposure, and the values for viral survival. In addition, the simplification of the presence of virus to a binary (yes/no), does not take into account viral load which is an important factor. Regardless, these assumptions are necessary for generating a conservative risk estimate because all assumptions made will lead to an overestimated probability of acquiring infection.

Third, estimates of the population level effect of infection acquisition were compromised by lack of data on the number of exposures. Infection control breaches may go unnoticed or unreported. In addition, estimates of the average number of exposures at the patient level are not available.

Fourth, reasons for syringe re-use by a HCW are seldom known - for example cost, time constraints, knowledge on the status of the patient (e.g., if the patient is known to be HIV or HCV positive, the HCW may avoid re-using the needle), and training may be contributing factors. Additionally, uncertainty surrounds the technique that the HCW uses to deliver the syringe content to the IV tubing; i.e., what factors determine a proximal vs. distal injection site, and does the HCW always verify line placement via blood return prior to administering the medication?

In conclusion, syringes are not meant to be re-used in health care settings in order to protect patient safety and guidelines were established in both Canada (1997) and the US (1995) to prevent this type of exposure. It is important to stress this message, especially when guidelines are not followed. Using a systematic tool to facilitate assessment of risk is very helpful in this regard. Thus, when there is a breach in practice guidelines or an outbreak of disease due to syringe re-use, quantitative risk assessments can provide estimates to help guide the response of regulators, public health officials and clinicians.

5. Acknowledgement

The authors thank Caroline Desjardins and Angela Catford for their assistance in preparing this manuscript. The authors also thank the referee for the invaluable comments and suggestions.

6. Appendix 1: Proofs of equations 1, 2 and 3

Proof of Equation 1

Let us suppress the dependence on year t for brevity in the following argument. Let k be the order of the patient among the s patients on which one syringe was used. If $k = 1$ then there is null risk on him/her. For each $k = 2, ..., s$, if the patient is not susceptible, there is also null risk on him/her. This patient will not contract the viral infection from any of the previous $k - 1$ patients if for each previous patient j, neither of the following happens:

1. carrying the virus,
2. transfer the virus to the syringe,
3. transmission happens to a patient after k-j re-uses

which has probability $\left(1 - Prev \times P^{(cont)} \times P_{k-j}^{(trans)}\right)$. Thus given that patient k is susceptible, by independence between the $k - 1$ patients the probability that the patient will not contract the viral infection from any of the previous $k - 1$ patients is $\prod_{j=1}^{k-1}\left(1 - Prev \times P^{(cont)} \times P_{k-j}^{(trans)}\right)$. Therefore, the probability of contracting the disease is

$$R_k = P^{(sus)} \times \left[1 - \prod_{j=1}^{k-1}\left(1 - Prev \times P^{(cont)} \times P_{k-j}^{(trans)}\right)\right].$$

Proof of Equation 2

Let us suppress the dependence on year t for brevity in the following argument. An individual chooses a national health care provider (HCP) that is practicing syringe re-use

(SR) with a probability $P(practice)$. If the selected HCP is practicing SR, then that individual can be uniformly any one of the group of S patients (S here is random since there is no guarantee of a specific system of SR) on which one syringe was re-used. So his/her probability of being any one of the group is $\frac{1}{S}$. Therefore, given that k is his/her order in the group, the probability of contracting a viral infection from any one of the previous $k - 1$ patients in the group is R_k.

Using the **Total Probability Rule,** the probability of acquiring the viral infection is given by

P(acquiring viral infection |practice done on S patients)

$$= \sum_{k=1}^{S} P(\text{acquiring viral infection |the patient's oreder among the S patients is k})$$

$$\times P(\text{the patient's oreder among the S patients is k}) = \sum_{k=1}^{S} R_k \times \frac{1}{S}.$$

Let $P(S = s)$ be the discrete probability distribution of the number of patients in one group. Using the **Total Probability Rule** one more time, the individual risk is given by

$$Risk = P(\text{acquiring viral infection |practice}) \times P(practice)$$
$$+ P(\text{acquiring viral infection |no practice}) \times (1 - P(practice)).$$

But P(acquiring viral infection |no practice) $= 0$. Hence,

$$Risk = P(\text{acquiring viral infection |practice}) \times P(practice)$$

and

$$P(\text{acquiring viral infection |practice}) = \sum_{s=2}^{\infty} P(\text{acquiring viral infection |practice done on S} = s) \times P(S = s) =$$

$$\sum_{s=2}^{\infty} \frac{1}{s} \sum_{k=1}^{S} R_k \times P(S = s).$$

Therefore,

$$Risk = P(practice) \times \sum_{s=2}^{\infty} \frac{1}{s} \sum_{k=1}^{S} R_k \times P(S = s).$$

Note that s starts from 2 since to have an SR practice it should be done on at least 2 patients in the one group and theoretically it can be on infinite number of patients but practically the sum will be truncated due to numerical negligence of the terms added.

Proof of Equation 3

Assuming that the nurse makes the decision of disposing the syringe randomly and independently of previous re-uses, the probabilistic experiment underlying the process is a geometric experiment. Let us also assume that the probability of syringe disposal (p) is independent of the number of elapsed re-uses and $M \geq 2$ be the average number of re-uses done in a HCP which need not to be an integer. Therefore, conditional that the number of re-uses of one syringe (or number patients in one group) S is at least 2, since we assume a SR practice; the mean would be given as

$$M = \sum_{s=2}^{\infty} s\, P(S = s) = \sum_{s=2}^{\infty} s \times p \times (1-p)^{s-2}$$

which implies that $p = \frac{1}{M-1}$.

Thus, the discrete probability distribution of the number of patients in one group is given by

$$P(S = s) = \frac{1}{M-1} \times \left(1 - \frac{1}{M-1}\right)^{s-2}$$

and equation (3) follows.

7. Appendix 2: Sensitivity analysis

The results of sensitivity analyses of the model output of the risk of HIV infection for several input variables for the proximal setting are shown in figure SI-1. This figure indicates that the model was most sensitive to uncertainty in the prevalence, followed by syringe re-use practice.

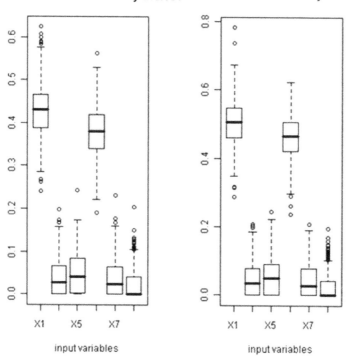

Fig. SI-1. First order sensitivity indices and total effects sensitivity indices for HIV infection risk in proximal setting scenario. *Legend*: X1 prevalence, X4 transmission, X5 contamination, X6 syringe re-use practice, and X7 the mean number of syringe re-use, and X8 log reduction.

Figure SI-2 shows the results of sensitivity analyses of the model output of the risk of HCV infection for several input variables for the proximal setting scenario. The figure shows the model was most sensitive to risk of transmission (X4), followed by the practice of syringe re-use (X6).

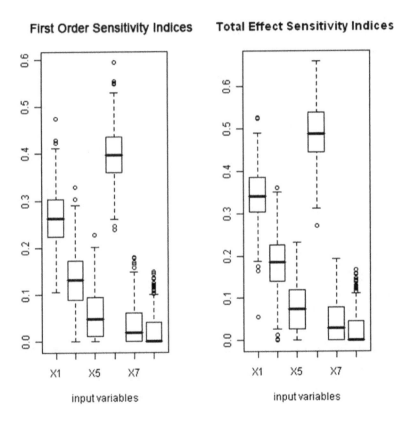

First Order Sensitivity Indices   Total Effect Sensitivity Indices

Fig. SI-2. First order sensitivity indices and total effects sensitivity indices for HCV infection risk in the proximal setting scenario. *Legend:* X1 prevalence, X4 transmission, X5 contamination, X6 syringe re-use practice, and X7 the mean number of syringe re-use, and X8 log reduction.

Figure SI-3 shows the first order sensitivity indices and total effects sensitivity indices for HBV infection risk in the proximal setting scenario. The individual risk was sensitive to prevalence (X1), transmission (X4), and practice of syringe re-use (X6).

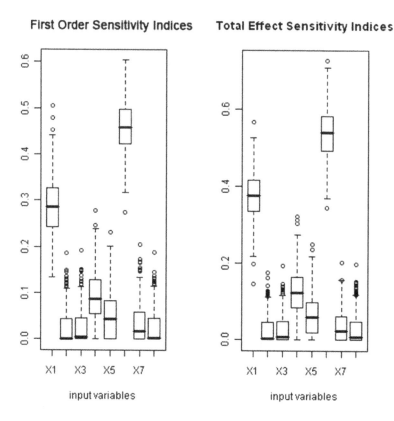

Fig. SI-3. First order sensitivity indices and total effects sensitivity indices for HBV infection risk in the proximal setting scenario. *Legend:* X1 prevalence, X2 immunized, X3 immunized but infected, X4 transmission, X5 contamination, X6 practice, X7 mean number of re-use, X8 log reduction.

Figure SI-4 shows the results of sensitivity analyses of the model output of the risk of HIV infection for several input variables for the distal setting (a scenario in which the syringe is re-used to inject drug in a site distal to the patient's IV set). As for the proximal setting, the model was sensitive for the prevalence (X1) and the practice of syringe re-use (X6).

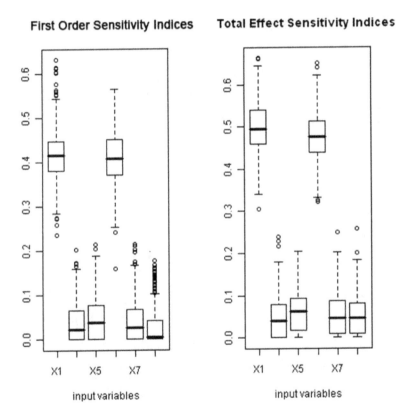

Fig. SI-4. First order sensitivity indices and total effects sensitivity indices for HIV infection risk in the distal setting scenario. *Legend:* X1 prevalence, X4 transmission, X5 contamination, X6 syringe re-use practice, and X7 the mean number of syringe re-use, and X8 log reduction.

Figure SI-5 shows the results of sensitivity analysis of the model output of the risk of HCV infection for several input variables for distal settings. The figure shows the model was most sensitive to uncertainty in the transmission (X4), followed the practice of syringe re-use (X6).

First Order Sensitivity Indices

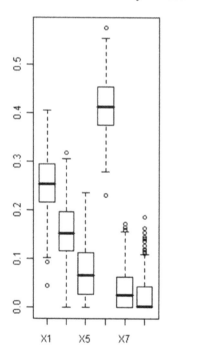

Total Effect Sensitivity Indices

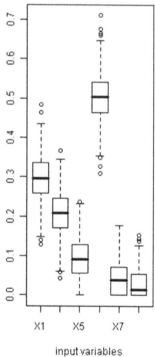

Fig. SI-5. First order sensitivity indices and total effects sensitivity indices for HCV infection risk in the distal setting scenario. *Legend*: X1 prevalence, X4 transmission, X5 contamination, X6 syringe re-use practice, and X7 the mean number of syringe re-use, and X8 log reduction.

Figure SI-6 shows the first order sensitivity indices and total effects sensitivity indices for HBV infection risk in the distal setting scenario. As for the proximal setting, the total effect was sensitive for prevalence (X1), transmission (X4), and practice of syringe re-use (X6).

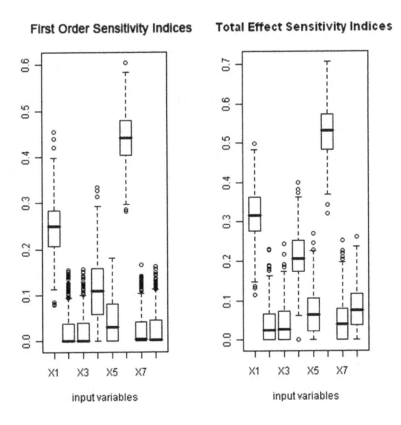

Fig. SI-6. The first order sensitivity indices and total effects sensitivity indices for HBV infection risk in the distal setting scenario. *Legend:* X1 prevalence, X2 immunized, X3 immunized but infected, X4 transmission, X5 contamination, X6 practice, X7 mean number of re-use, X8 log reduction.

8. References

American Society of Anesthesiologists 1999, Recommendations for Infection Control for the Practice of Anesthesiology 2nd Edition.

CBC News-Edmonton, 10-31-2008a. Saskatchewan hospital also reused syringes: health officials, CBC News.

CBC News-Edmonton, 10-31-2008b. Syringe reuse might be happening across Canada: Alberta health official, CBC News.

Government of Alberta. (3-19-2009. Provincial review of infection control practices complete.

Gramacy, R. & Taddy, M. Bayesian treed Gaussian process models (tgp)- R package. 2009.
Ref Type: Computer Program

Lessard, M.R., Trepanier, C.A., Gourdeau, M., & Denault, P.H. 1988. A microbiological study of the contamination of the syringes used in anaesthesia practice. Can.J.Anaesth., 35, (6) 567-569

Mackie, C.O., Buxton, J.A., Tadwalkar, S., & Patrick, D.M. 2009. Hepatitis B immunization strategies: timing is everything. CMAJ., 180, (2) 196-202

Perceval, A. 1980. Consequence of syringe-plunger contamination. Med.J.Aust., 1, (10) 487-489

Population Health Branch-Saskatchewan Health 2009, Assessing risk from syringe reuse in Saskatchewan.

Public Health Agency of Canada 2006, The Canadian Immunization Guide 7th edition.

Public Health Agency of Canada. (11-4-2008. Canada's Chief Public Health Officer stresses the importance of infection control practices.

Public Health Agency of Canada. 2009, Internal documentation: Risk Assessment Model to Determine the Risk of Viral Infection Due to Improper Re-use of Syringes, Commissioned expert working group.

R Development Core Team. R: A Language and Environment for Statistical Computing. 2010. Vienna, Austria, R Foundation for Statistical Computing. 2009.
Ref Type: Computer Program

Sikora, C., Chandran, A.U., Joffe, A.M., Johnson, D., & Johnson, M. 2010. Population Risk of Syringe Reuse: Estimating the Probability of Transmitting Bloodborne Disease. Infection Control and Hospital Epidemiology, 31, (7) 748-754 available from: ISI:000278374000013

Part 2

Health Risk Assessment Case Studies for Emerging Risks

Ultrafine and Fine Aerosol Deposition in the Nasal Airways of a 9-Month-Old Girl, a 5-Year-Old Boy and a 53-Year-Old Male

Jinxiang Xi[1,2], JongWon Kim[1] and Xiuhua A. Si[3]
[1]University of Arkansas at Little Rock, Little Rock, AR,
[2]Central Michigan University, Mount Pleasant, MI
[3]Calvin College, Grand Rapids, MI,
USA

1. Introduction

Exposure to environmental aerosols of submicrometer size may cause significant risks to human health. Submicrometer aerosols include particles in the ultrafine (<100 nm) and fine (100 nm to 1 μm) regimes. Recent studies indicate that aerosols in this size range are biologically more active and potentially more toxic than micrometer particles of the same material (Kreyling et al., 2006; Kreyling et al., 2004; Li et al., 2003; Oberdorster and Utell 2002). Sources of submicrometer aerosols include diesel exhaust (50 to 500 nm) (Kittelson 1998), cigarette smoke (140 to 500 nm) (Bernstein 2004; Keith 1982), and radioactive decay (1 to 200 nm) (ICRP 1994). Submicrometer bioaerosols include respiratory specific viruses such as Avian flu and SARS, which typically range from 20 to 200 nm (Mandell et al., 2004). These aerosols may deposit in the respiratory airways in discrete amounts resulting in local injury and spread of infectious diseases. Considering the extrathoracic nasal airways, which include the nasal passages, pharynx, and larynx, the deposition of submicrometer aerosols is associated with a number of detrimental health effects. The deposition of cigarette smoke particles has been quantitatively linked to the formation of respiratory tract tumors at specific sites (Martonen 1986). Yang et al. (1989) reported that respiratory tract cancers per unit surface area are approximately 3,000 times more likely in the extrathoracic airways including the larynx. Ostiguy et al. (2008) summarized the adverse health effects due to various nanoparticles such as carbon nanotubes, fullerenes, inorganic and organic nanoparticles, and quantum dots. Gurr *et al.* (2005) studied the effect of ultrafine TiO2 particles on human bronchial epithelial cells and reported that TiO2 particles of 10 and 20 nm triggered oxidative DNA damage and lipid peroxidation, the later of which may also explains the cytotoxicity of water-soluble fullerenes or nC60 (Sayes *et al.*, 2005).

Compared to adults, infants and children are more susceptible to respiratory risks. Exposure to ambient toxicants in children may cause adverse effects such as nasal obstruction, sinusitis, nasal carcinomas, and spread of infectious diseases. Respiratory disease remains a leading cause of childhood morbidity in the U.S. and other developed countries and is a leading cause to childhood deaths worldwide (U.S. Surgeon General Report 2007). Epidemiological studies have shown that children are biologically more susceptible to particulate matters (PM) than adults due to their immature defense mechanism and detoxification pathways (U.S. Surgeon General Report 2007). Besides, children usually spend more time outdoors, breath faster, and therefore may receive a greater dose of PM than adults. Those children with a history of asthma often exhibit elevated levels of other respiratory symptoms such as cough, bronchitis, or pneumonia when living in highly polluted areas (California EPA 2005). Passive tobacco smoke exposure can also cause different health problems. Specifically, it (1) increases the frequency and severity of children's cold, sore throat, and asthma, (2) aggravates sinusitis, rhinitis, cystic fibrosis, and chronic respiratory problems, and (3) causes recurrent ear infections (California EPA 2005).

In contrast with potentially negative health effects, inhalation therapy for infants and children has been employed to deliver pharmaceutical aerosols to the lung via nasal route or to the nasal passages as the direct target. Aerosol delivery issues specific to children include lower tidal volumes, smaller airway size, and use of mask versus mouthpiece. Only a small amount of the applied dose reaches the target receptor in children. Studies have shown that for adults about 10% of the administered drug reaches the lung whereas for infants and toddlers this percentage is usually less than 1% (Everard 2003). Therefore, children adapted methods, dose, and devices are likely to increase therapeutic options leading to improved inhalation therapy and medical outcomes.

A number of *in vivo* and *in vitro* studies have considered the deposition of submicrometer aerosols in the nasal airway. *In vitro* studies that evaluated the nasal deposition of ultrafine aerosols in humans include Cheng et al. (1996a) and Swift and Strong (1996). The study of Cheng et al. (1996a) considered the deposition of aerosols ranging from 4 – 150 nm in 10 subjects and quantified variability in nasal geometries using MRI scans. Deposition was shown to be a function of nasal cavity surface area, minimum cross-sectional area, and shape complexity. *In vitro* studies provide the advantage of avoiding human subject testing and can determine depositions within specific regions of the nasal cavity. A number of *in vitro* studies have considered deposition of ultrafine aerosols in replicas of human noses (Cheng 2003; Cheng et al., 1993; Cheng et al., 1988; Gradon and Yu 1989; Guilmette et al., 1994; Kelly et al., 2004b; Yamada et al., 1988). The nasal geometries used in these studies are typically derived from medical scan data (CT and MRI) or casts of cadavers. Results of the available *in vitro* experiments are in general agreement with the deposition data from *in vivo* studies for ultrafine aerosols (Cheng et al., 1996a). Based on a collection of *in vivo* nasal deposition studies, Cheng et al. (1996b) suggested a best-fit correlation for particle sizes less than 150 nm. Later, Cheng et al. (2003) incorporated *in vivo* and *in vitro* nasal deposition data of ultrafine and micrometer particles to develop a correlation for particle sizes in the diffusional and the impaction deposition regimes. A common disadvantage of both *in vivo* and *in vitro* methods is the difficulty in determining local deposition values.

Previous numerical studies have considered the transport and deposition of fine and ultrafine particles in the nasal cavity (Liu et al., 2007; Martonen et al., 2003; Schroeter et al., 2001; Shi et al., 2006; Xi and Longest 2008; Xi and Longest 2009; Yu et al., 1998; Zamankhan et al., 2006). Similar CFD studies have also evaluated the transport and absorption of dilute chemical species in the nasal passages (Cohen Hubal et al., 1996; Scherer et al., 1994; Zhao et al., 2004). Compared with *in vitro* and *in vivo* studies, CFD predictions have the advantage of providing detailed information on airflow and aerosol deposition, like hot spots that are more relevant to health outcome than the average deposition. However, to the authors' knowledge, very few CFD studies have been reported so far studying children nasal

Ultrafine and Fine Aerosol Deposition in the Nasal Airways of a 9-Month-Old Girl, a 5-Year-Old Boy and
a 53-Year-Old Male

33

depositions, with one exception being Xi et al. (2011) that examined the transport and depositions of micrometer particles. The general neglect of child or infant nasal airways in previous studies may largely attribute to limited accessibility of pediatric medical images to CFD practitioners as well as the complexities involved in constructing physiologically realistic nasal passages. Concerning the age-related effect, several investigators have evaluated lung depositions of micrometer aerosols using scaled-down tracheobronchial models representative of growing lungs at different ages (Asgharian et al., 2004; Crawford 1982; Oldham et al., 1997; Xu and Yu 1986). In these studies, significant variations in micrometer particle lung deposition with respect to age were observed, with higher deposition in children than adults. However, no numerical study has considered the age-related effects upon the nasal deposition of ultrafine and fine-regime aerosols.

The objective of this chapter is to assess the age effects on airflow and aerosol dynamics within the nasal cavity in a systemic manner. There are three specific goals in this study: (1) quantifying morphologic dimensions of the nasal airway models for a 9-month-old girl, a 5-year-old boy, and a 53-year-old adult; (2) numerically characterizing the breathing resistance, airflow dynamics, and particle transport within the nasal passages during inhalation; and (3) numerically evaluating the deposition of submicrometer aerosols in the infant, child, and adult nasal airways on a total, sub-regional, and localized basis. Results of this study may lead to a better understanding of the developmental respiratory physiology and the associated effects on children's health response to environmental pollutants, or the medical outcome from inhalation therapy for infants and children.

Parameter	Range
d_p (nm)	Ultrafine: 1, 2, 3, 5, 10, 20, 50, 100
	Fine: 100, 200, 300, 400, 500, 700, 1,000
Flow rate Q_{in} (L/min)	3, 5, 7.5, 10, 15, 20, 30, 45
Cunningham correction factor C_c	221 – 1.15
Particle diffusivity $\tilde{D}$ (cm²/s)	$5.44 \times 10^{-2} - 2.84 \times 10^{-7}$
Schmidt number $Sc = \nu / \tilde{D}$	$2.92 - 5.61 \times 10^{-5}$
Particle Stokes number St_k	$2.4 \times 10^{-8} - 3.0 \times 10^{-3}$
Flow Reynolds number at the inlet	189 – 5,243

Table 1. Test conditions for the three airway models

2. Methods

To achieve the above goals, anatomically realistic nasal airway models have been constructed based on CT/MRI images. Breathing scenarios ranging from sedentary through heavy activity conditions (i.e., 3–30 L/min) and inhaled particles ranging from 1 nm to 1,000 nm are considered (Table 1). Details of the geometry construction, inhalation conditions, and particle transport models are described below.

2.1 Construction of the nasal airway models

For inhalation toxicology and pharmaceutical research, imaged-based modeling represents a significant improvement compared with conventional cadaver casting, which is subject to distortion due to the shrinkage of mucous membranes or insertion of casting materials. Pritchard and McRobbie (2004) compared a cadaver cast with their MRI oropharyngeal airway model averaged over 20 subjects (10 males and 10 females) and showed significant geometric disparities. The most prominent difference was the greater volume of the cadaver casts, which was 92.7 cm³ for the cast versus 46.7 cm³ (SD12.7) for imaging. Generally, a physical model produced from anatomical images results in about 5% difference in the airway volume and some loss of fine morphological details. Therefore, this approach may adequately approximate the internal geometries (Pritchard and McRobbie 2004).

(a) MRI/CT   (b) Solid Body   (c) Defining Polylines   (d) Surface Model   (e) Mesh

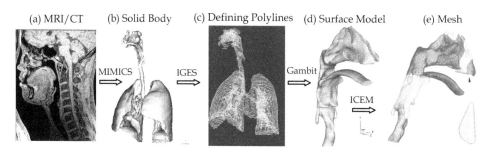

Fig. 1. Procedures of 3D rendering of CT/MRI images.

We will use one example to illustrate the computer method for developing a surface model of the respiratory tract based on medical images such as CT or MRI data. Figures 1a–e illustrate the procedure of translating from CT scans into a high-quality computational mesh of the nasal-laryngeal airway (Xi et al. 2010). To construct the 3D airway model, CT scans of a healthy non-smoking 53-year-old male (weight 73 kg and height 173 cm) were used, which were obtained with a multirow-detector helical CT scanner (GE medical systems, Discovery LS) and the following acquisition parameters: 0.7 mm effective slice spacing, 0.65 mm overlap, 1.2 mm pitch, and 512×512 pixel resolution. The multi-slice CT images were then imported into MIMICS (Materialise, Ann Arbor MI) and were segmented according to the contrast between osseous structures and intra-airway air to convert the raw image data into a set of cross-sectional contours that define the solid geometry (Figs. 1a–c). Based on these contours, a surface geometry was constructed in Gambit 2.3 (Ansys, Inc.) (Fig. 1d). The surface geometry was then imported into ANSYS ICEM (Ansys, Inc.) as an IGES file for meshing. Due to the high complexity of the model geometry, an unstructured tetrahedral mesh was created with high-resolution pentahedral elements in the near-wall region (Fig. 1e). The main geometric features retained in this example include nasal passages, nasopharynx (NP), pharynx, and throat. In particular, anatomical details such as uvula, epiglottal fold, and laryngeal sinus are retained. The resulting model is intended to faithfully represent the anatomy of the extrathoracic airway with only minor surface smoothing. Similarly, MRI scans of a healthy 5-year-old boy (weight 21 kg and height 109 cm) and CT scans of a 9-month-old girl (weight and height unknown) were used in this study to construct the pediatric nasal airway models. In order to quantitatively evaluate the flow field and aerosol depositions within the nasal airway, the airway model is divided into different sections (Fig. 2). In the main flow direction, subregions include the nasal vestibule and valve region (V&V), turbinate region (TR), nasopharynx (NP), pharynx and larynx. On top of the nasal airway is the olfactory region (OR) where the sensory nerves are located.

Ultrafine and Fine Aerosol Deposition in the Nasal Airways of a 9-Month-Old Girl, a 5-Year-Old Boy and a 53-Year-Old Male

35

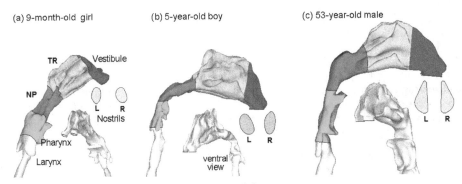

Fig. 2. Image-based nasal-laryngeal airway models.

2.2 Boundary conditions

Steady inhalation was assumed for all simulations with uniform velocity profiles at both nose inlets (nostrils) (Fig. 2). Initial particle velocities were assumed to be the same as the local fluid velocity. The airway surface was assumed to be smooth and rigid with no-slip (u_{wall} = 0) and perfect absorption conditions. In the body, the extrathoracic airway is covered with a thin layer of mucus, which captures particles at initial contact and clears them to the throat or nasal vestibule by mucocilliary movement within a time period of 10 to 15 minutes. Mass diffusion and metabolism of deposited particles may occur within the mucus layer and may change the zero-concentration conditions at the wall. However, due to the slow speed of the mucocilliary movement compared with the intranasal airflow and relatively low deposition rates, the no-slip and perfect absorption conditions are reasonable approximations in this study.

2.3 Fluid and particle dynamics equations

Flows in this study are assumed to be isothermal and incompressible. The mean inlet Reynolds number at the trachea varies from 368 to 3,302. The maximum Reynolds number based on the hydraulic diameter of the glottal aperture is approximately 8,037. Multi-regime flow dynamics can coexist in the nasal airway due to its unique physiology. To resolve the possible laminar-transitional-turbulent flow conditions, the low Reynolds number (LRN) k-ω model was selected based on its ability to accurately predict pressure drop, velocity profiles, and shear stress for transitional and turbulent flows. Moreover, the LRN k-ω model was shown to provide an accurate solution for laminar flow as the turbulent viscosity approaches zero (Wilcox 1998).

The transport and deposition of the submicrometer particles are simulated with a well-tested discrete Lagrangian tracking model enhanced with near-wall treatment. The aerosols evaluated in this study had a density of 1.0 g/cm³ and particle Stokes number ($St_k = \rho_p d_p^2 U/18\mu D_h$) range of 0.00001 to 1.0. The inhaled particles were assumed to be dilute and had no influence upon the continuous-phase, i.e., one-way coupled particle motion. In our previous studies, the Lagrangian tracking model enhanced with user-defined routines was shown to provide close agreement with experimental deposition data in upper respiratory airways for both submicrometer (Xi et al., 2008) and micrometer particles (Xi and Longest 2007). The discrete Lagrangian transport equations can be expressed as

$$\frac{dv_i}{dt} = \alpha \frac{Du_i}{Dt} + \frac{f}{\tau_p}(u_i - v_i) + g_i(1 - \alpha) + f_{i,Brownian} \quad \text{and} \quad \frac{dx_i}{dt} = v_i(t) \tag{1}$$

where v_i and u_i are the components of the particle and local fluid velocity, and τ_p (i.e., ρ_p $d_p^2/18\mu$) is the characteristic time required for a particle to respond to changes in the flow field. The drag factor f, which represents the ratio of the drag coefficient C_D to Stokes drag, is based on the expression of Morsi and Alexander (1972). The influence of non-uniform fluctuations in the near-wall region is taken into account by implementing an anisotropic turbulence model proposed by Matida et al. (2004), which is described as

$$u'_n = f_v \xi \sqrt{2k/3} \quad and \quad f_v = 1 - \exp(-0.002y^+) \tag{2}$$

In this equation, ξ is a random number generated from a Gaussian probability density function and f_v is a damping function component normal to the wall for values of y^+ less than 40. Away from the wall ($y^+ > 40$), $f_v = 1$.

Evaluation of the particle trajectory equation requires that the fluid velocity u_i be determined at the particle location for each time-step. On a computational grid, determining the fluid velocity at the particle location requires spatial interpolation from control-volume centers or nodal values. Based on studies of deposition in the oral airway using Fluent 6, fluid velocities in wall-adjacent control volumes were observed to maintain the value at the control-volume center and not approach zero at the wall (Longest and Xi 2007). Longest and Xi (2007) reported that a near-wall interpolation (NWI) algorithm provided an effective approach to accurately predict the deposition of nanoparticles in the respiratory tract. A user-defined routine was developed that linearly interpolates the fluid velocity in near-wall control-volumes from nodal values. Velocity values at the wall were taken to be zero.

2.4 Numerical method and convergence sensitivity analysis

To solve the governing mass and momentum conservation equations in each of the cases considered, the CFD package ANSYS Fluent 6.3 was employed. User-supplied Fortran and C programs were implemented for the calculations of inlet flow and particle profiles, particle transport and deposition locations, grid convergence, and deposition enhancement factors. A specific set of user-defined functions was also applied for implementing the anisotropic turbulence effect and near-wall velocity interpolation. All transport equations were discretized to be at least second order accurate in space. A segregated implicit solver was employed to evaluate the resulting linear system of equations. This solver uses the Gauss-Seidel method in conjunction with an algebraic multigrid approach for improving the calculation performance on tetrahedral meshes. Convergence of the flow field solution was assumed when the global mass residual was reduced from its original value by five orders of magnitude and when the residual-reduction-rates for both mass and momentum were sufficiently small.

The computational meshes of the four nasal-laryngeal airway models were generated with ANSYS ICEM 12.0 (Ansys, Inc.). An unstructured tetrahedral mesh was generated with high-resolution prismatic cells in the near-wall region (Fig. 3) to accommodate the high complexity of the model geometry. A grid sensitivity analysis was conducted by testing the effects of different mesh densities with approximately 540,200, 980,900, 1,750,000 and

2,812,000 control volumes while keeping the near-wall cell height constant at 0.05 mm (Xi et al., 2008). Increasing grid resolution from 1,750,000 to 2,812,000 control volumes resulted in total deposition changes of less than 1%. As a result, the final grid for reporting flow field and deposition conditions consisted of approximately 1,750,000 cells with a thin five-layer pentahedral grid in the near-wall region and a first near-wall cell height of 0.05 mm.

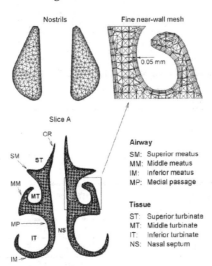

Fig. 3. Coronal view of the ICEM-generated computational mesh of the 53-year-old male.

For discrete Lagrangian tracking, the number of seeded particles required to produce count-independent depositions was tested. Particle count sensitivity analysis was performed by incrementally releasing groups of 10,000 particles. The number of groups was increased until the deposition rate changed by < 1%. The final number of particles tracked for ultrafine and fine-regime aerosols were 60,000 and 100,000 respectively.

3. Results

3.1 Infant-child-adult discrepancy

The differences of nasal airways among a 9-month-old girl, a 5-year-old boy (Xi et al., 2011) and a 53-year-old male reported previously (Xi and Longest 2008) are quite obvious in both morphology and dimensions. As for the morphology, younger subjects have smaller sized nostrils, shorter turbinate regions, longer but thinner nasopharynx, and thinner pharynx-larynx. It is therefore expected that as a human grows from birth to adulthood, the airway geometry keeps changing, which in turn alters the nasal aerodynamics as well as the deposition patterns of inhaled aerosols.

A quantitative comparison of airway dimensions among these three subjects is shown in Fig. 4 in terms of coronal cross-sectional area and hydraulic diameter d_h, both as a function of distance from the nose tip. Comparison of airway volume and surface area among the three subjects for various nasal anatomical sections are listed in Table 2. The dimension of two nostrils and upper trachea are shown in Table 3. It is noted that the test conditions (such as geographical elevation) are not clear for these three subjects, and the differences

Anatomical sections*	Volume, V (cm³)			Surface area, A (cm²)			Effective diameter, d_e‡ (cm)		
	9-m	5-yr	Adult	9-m	5-yr	Adult	9-m	5-yr	Adult
V&V	1.25	3.37	5.50	9.75	23.74	35.58	0.512	0.568	0.619
TR	2.83	11.03	12.63	35.63	107.34	112.59	0.318	0.411	0.449
NP	1.74	3.95	16.33	9.27	15.27	40.93	0.750	1.034	1.595
Pharynx	3.19	2.64	13.89	13.71	14.59	45.10	0.932	0.724	1.232
Larynx	1.32	1.22	6.70	8.37	7.20	21.81	0.629	0.676	1.228
Total	10.33	22.21	55.05	76.73	168.14	256.01	0.538	0.528	0.860

* V&V (vestibule and valve region), TR (turbinate region), NP (nasopharynx)
‡ Effective diameter $d_e = 4V/A$

Table 2. Comparison of nasal airway dimension among an infant, a child and an adult.

Anatomical sections	Cross-sect area, A (mm²)			Perimeter, P (mm)			Hydr. diameter, d_h‡ (mm)		
	9-m	5-yr	Adult	9-m	5-yr	Adult	9-m	5-yr	Adult
R nostril	27.98	49.20	101.27	19.92	25.61	44.53	5.62	7.68	9.10
L nostril	31.48	43.74	101.27	20.49	24.89	44.53	6.15	7.03	9.10
Trachea	50.64	83.23	148.66	25.59	33.59	45.66	8.01	9.91	13.02

‡ Hydraulic diameter $d_h = 4A/P$

Table 3. Dimension of the nostrils and upper trachea of the three airway models.

presented herein are assumed to be mainly attributed to the age effect. From Table 2, the nasal airway volume of the 9-month-old infant and the 5-year-old child is 18.8% and 40.3% that of the adult, respectively; while the nasal airway surface area of the infant and child is 30.0% and 65.7% that of the adult, respectively. In particular, two major disparities are noted. First, the infant and child both possess a much narrower and smaller nasopharynx lumen compared to that of the adult. From Fig. 4a, the NP cross-sectional area of the infant (i.e., A = 78 mm²) and child (i.e., A = 170 mm²) is only one seventh and one third that of the adult (i.e., A = 535 mm²) respectively. From Fig. 4c, the NP hydraulic diameter of the infant (i.e., 8.1 mm) and the child (i.e., d_h = 12.2 mm) is about one third and half that of the adult (i.e., d_h = 24.0 mm), respectively. Secondly, the distance to the nasal valve (the minimum cross-sectional area) is much shorter for the 9-month infant (11.2 mm, blue solid arrow in Fig. 4a) compared to the 5-year-old child (20.8 mm, black arrow) and adult (27.2 mm, red arrow). Similarly, the nasal valve area is also much smaller for the infant (i.e., ~56 mm²) compared to both the child and adult, while the later two subjects have similar valve areas (i.e., ~180 mm²) (Fig. 4a). This observation may imply that the nasal valve matures at early ages (around 5 years old). Another similar observation is for the nasal turbinate region, where the hydraulic diameter of the child and adult are very close (~10.0 mm) while that of the infant is much smaller (~3.8 mm).

Ultrafine and Fine Aerosol Deposition in the Nasal Airways of a 9-Month-Old Girl, a 5-Year-Old Boy and
a 53-Year-Old Male

39

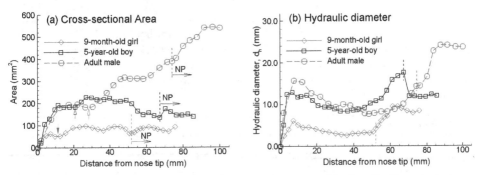

Fig. 4. Comparison of nasal cross-sectional area, perimeter, and hydraulic diameter between
a 9-month-old girl, a five-year-old boy, and an adult male.

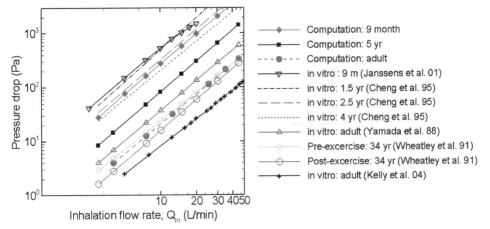

Fig. 5. Pressure drop (i.e., breathing impedance) as a function of inhalation flow rate with
comparison to *in vitro* and *in vivo* measurements in various age groups.

3.2 Breathing resistance

Figure 5 shows the predicted breathing resistance (Δp) within the infant, child, and adult
nasal airways considered in this study in comparison with existing *in vitro* and *in vivo*
measurements for various age groups. *In vitro* data presented include an infant (9 month)
(Janssens et al., 2001), young children (1.5 yr, 2.5 yr, 4 yr) (Cheng et al., 1995c), and adults
(Kelly et al., 2004a; Yamada et al., 1988). *In vivo* data are from adult subjects (34 ± 5 yr)
before and after exercise (Wheatley et al., 1991). In general, the pressure drop (i.e., breathing
impedance) decreases as the age increases. Infants and children have much higher breathing
impedance than adults for a same flow rate. As expected, the pressure drop curve of the 9-
month infant agrees fairly well with the 9-month *in vitro* measurements (Janssens et al.,
2001), and that of the 5-year-old boy falls between those of young children and adults.
Children grow fast in height and weight before the age of seven and the rate of growth
decreases thereafter, so does the growth of nasal airway. It is therefore reasonable that the
infant breathing resistance is much higher while the 5-year-old breathing resistance is

somewhat between infants and adults. The pressure-flow relationships can be expressed as a power function ($\Delta P = a \cdot Q^b$), which can be plotted as straight lines on a log-log scale with slope "b". Table 4 lists the coefficients "a" and "b" for subjects of different ages. In light of the age-related effects, "a" constantly decreases in magnitude as age increases (from 8.87 at 9 month old to 0.54–0.16 when grown up) whereas the slopes of the Δp-Q_{in} curve are similar for all ages (b = 1.71–1.98).

Age/Reference	Method	a^*	b^*
9 m (Saint), Janssens (01)	*in vitro*, CT cast	8.87	1.75
9 m, This study	CFD, CT model	4.01	1.84
1.5 yr, Cheng (95)	*in vitro*, MRI cast	5.24±0.70	1.98±0.060
2.5 yr, Cheng (95)	*in vitro*, MRI cast	4.46±0.15	1.87±0.014
4 yr, Cheng (95)	*in vitro*, MRI cast	3.40±0.20	1.86±0.023
5 yr, This study	CFD, MRI model	1.07	1.89
Adult, Yamada (88)	*in vitro*, Cadaver cast	0.54	1.85
34 ± 5 yr, Wheatley (95)	*in vivo*, Pre-exercise	0.43±0.34	1.75±0.030
34 ± 5 yr, Wheatley (95)	*in vivo*, Post-exercise	0.20±0.35	1.90±0.028
53 yr, This study	CFD, MRI model	0.31	1.84
53 yr, Kelly (04)	*in vitro*, MRI cast, (nose only)	0.16	1.71

$* \Delta P (Pa) = aQ (L / \min)^b$

Table 4. Pressure drop (i.e., breathing impedance) in nasal airways at different ages,

3.3 Airflow field and particle transport

Comparison of airflow fields in the infant, child, and adult nasal airways are shown in Fig. 6 for an inhalation flow rate of 20 L/min. It is noted that this flow rate represents quite different physical activity conditions for the three subjects, i.e., light activity for the adult, medium activity for the child, and heavy activity for the infant. It is also noted that different velocity scale is used in each model. From Fig. 6, flows of high velocity magnitude are observed in the middle portion of the nasal passage for all the three models considered. In contrast, the narrow fin-like meatus regions receive a minimal fraction of the airflow, especially in the deeper portions of each meatus. The main flow changes its direction dramatically from the nostrils to the nasopharynx, forming a nearly 180° curvature; however, this curvature is less severe for the infant model compared to the other two, preassembly resulting from a more back-tilted head position of the infant during image acquiring. No recirculation zone is observed in the infant and child NP due to a much smaller airway diameter in this region, which is different from the adult NP where flow recirculation is obvious (Xi and Longest 2008).

To compare secondary velocity motions of the three models considered, two-dimensional stream traces are plotted in the anterior and posterior passages of each model (Slices 2-2' and 3-3'). Due to the thin air channels, vortices are damped and not discernable in the nasal passage. The magnitude of the secondary velocity in each slice is approximately 10% - 30% of the main flow. It is interesting to note that the relative strength of the second motion

Ultrafine and Fine Aerosol Deposition in the Nasal Airways of a 9-Month-Old Girl, a 5-Year-Old Boy and a 53-Year-Old Male

41

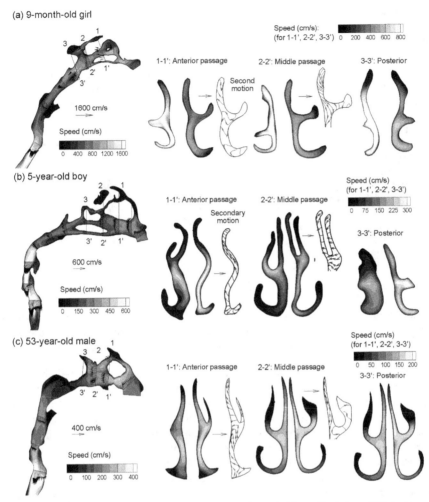

Fig. 6. Velocity fields in the nasal passages of the infant, child, and adult at 20L/min.

varies among the three age groups, which progressively increases as age increases. Take the middle passage (Slice 2-2') as an example. The ratio of the secondary velocity to the mean speed is 3.6 to 25% with a median of 16% for the 9-month infant, 9.8 - 36% with a median of 25% for the 5-year-old child, and 13 to 40% with a median of 29% for the adult. The secondary motion functions to distribute the inhaled air into each fin-like meatus. Therefore, this difference might reflect the more matured (and more complicated) nasal turbinate at elder ages that more effectively convey the airflow throughout the nasal passages. Of particular interest is the observation of transportation of airflow toward the olfactory region. The secondary flows move upward prior to the olfactory region (Slice 2-2') and downward after the olfactory region (Slice 3-3'). It is expected that the secondary motion near the olfactory region is delicately balanced, which should be large enough to convey a sufficient amount of particles or vapors for the olfactory nerve to perceive while still remaining small enough to protect this extremely sensitive area that is directly connected to the brain. It is also interesting to note that the right and left nasal passages are quite different both in geometry and flow fields for all the three models considered, with one passage being more constricted than the other (Fig. 6). This geometric disparity is possibly attributed to the natural nasal cycle during which the airway obstruction alternates over a period of several hours (Eccles 1996). The resulting difference in airflows between the right and left passages has been suggested to help the central nerve system to locate where smell comes from.

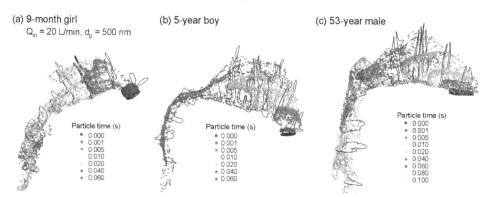

Fig. 7. Snapshots of particle locations through the right nasal passage of (a) 9-month-old girl, (b) 5-year-old boy, and (c) 53-year-old male. For each model, an amount of 2,000 particles of 500 nm were released at the right nostril at t = 0 ms and recorded at various instants.

Particle transport within the right nasal passage of the three models considered are visualized in Fig. 7 as snapshots of particle locations at specified instants for an inhalation flow rate of 20 L/min. Two thousand 500 nm particles were released at the right nostril at t = 0 ms and particle positions were recorded after designated period of times. Due to the small inertia and diffusion of the aerosols considered, particles are assumed to closely follow the airflow. For all the three models, faster transport and deeper penetration of aerosols are apparent in the medial passages while slow-moving particles are found near the airway walls. Because of the dramatic airway bend from the nostril to the nasopharynx, a high-concentration of particles constantly adjusts their directions following the mean streamline curvature of inhaled airflows. Considering that 20 L/min represents different levels of physical activity for the three subjects considered, the time required for the aerosols to fill the nasal airway also varies. It takes about 20 ms for particles to first reach the upper trachea for the infant (green symbols), whereas it takes 60 ms for the child, and 100 ms for the adult. The seemingly random particle distributions downstream of the nasopharynx indicate enhanced turbulent mixing in those regions. Due to the small-sized nasopharynx-larynx in both the infant and child, particles in this region are transported at a much higher rate than in adult (i.e., from NP to larynx taking 10 ms for the infant, 20 ms for the child, vs. 40 ms for the adult).

3.4 Particle deposition

Comparison of surface depositions in the infant, child, and adult nasal airways are shown in Fig. 8 for aerosols within both ultrafine (1–10 nm) and fine (100–1,000 nm) regimes at a constant inhalation flow rate of 20 L/min. Overall, much similarity than difference was

Ultrafine and Fine Aerosol Deposition in the Nasal Airways of a 9-Month-Old Girl, a 5-Year-Old Boy and a 53-Year-Old Male

43

observed in the three models considered, whose deposition patterns exhibit much less heterogeneity than that we observed for micron particles (Xi et al., 2011). As expected, a large amount of ultrafine aerosols deposit in the nasal airways for all the models considered, while only a small amount of fine-regime aerosols deposit. In light of local depositions, ultrafine aerosols accumulate either in turbinate region or pharynx-larynx region, while the fine-regime aerosols accumulate mainly in the pharynx-larynx region where turbulence is most pronounced. One explanation for the ultrafine particle accumulation in the turbinate region is the narrow airway channel with the high particle diffusivity that disperses ultrafine particles onto the turbinate walls.

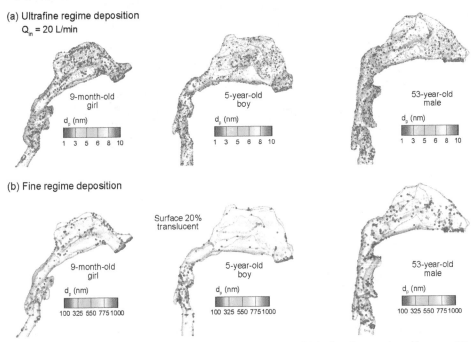

Fig. 8. Surface deposition in the three models of particles of (a) ultrafine regime (1 nm to 10 nm only) and (b) fine regime (100 nm to 1,000 nm). The fine-regime depositions are shown with 50% translucence.

Figure 9 shows the 3-D surface plot of the deposition fractions in the infant, child, and adult nasal airways as a function of both inhalation flow rate and particle size. The inhalation flow rates considered are 3, 5, 7.5, 10, 15, 20, 30, 45 L/min and the particle sizes are in the range of 1–1,000 nm. The three surface plots look alike both in trend and magnitude, with declining deposition rate as the particle size and flow speed increase. The peak deposition rate occurs at the smallest particle size and lowest flow rate considered (d_p = 1 nm and Q_{in} = 3 L/min) where the Brownian motion and residence time of the particles are both maximal. However, the relative role of the convective (flow rate) and molecular (particle size) diffusion differs in the ultrafine aerosol deposition, as the effect of molecular diffusion apparently overweighs that of convection for the breathing conditions considered herein. Considering the fine regime particles in the range of 100–1,000 nm, very low deposition fractions are observed for all models considered. However, further examination of Fig. 9 reveals an interesting phenomenon associated with the interactions between mechanisms of diffusion and inertial impaction. For all three models considered, the deposition rate decreases first and then starts to increase with increasing particle size and flow rate. This valley-shaped profile results from a competition between the diminishing diffusive effect and enlarging finite inertial effect as the particle size and flow rate continuously rise, with the minimum occurring when the sum of these two effects is the smallest. But the breathing scenario of minimal deposition varies for the three age groups, which is at the inhalation flow rate of ~3 L/min for the infant and child, and is ~10 L/min for the adult, as shown in Fig. 9.

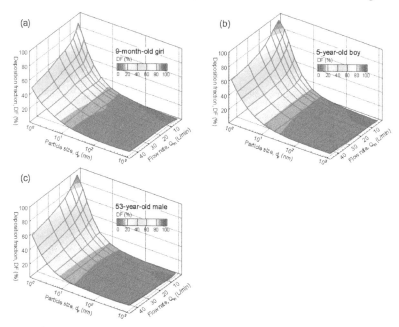

Fig. 9. 3-D surface plot of the total deposition fractions as a function of particle diameter and inhalation flow rate in the nasal-laryngeal airway models of (a) 9-month-old girl, (b) 5-year-old boy, and (c) 53-year-old male.

To further evaluate the predicted deposition results, the same data set from Fig. 9 has been plotted as a function of two existing diffusion parameters proposed from *in vitro* and *in vivo* deposition studies (Fig. 10). The first parameter ($D^{0.5}Q^{-0.125}$) was theoretically derived by Cheng et al. (1988) based on the assumption of turbulent diffusion in pipe flow and was later adopted in a series of *in vitro* replica studies (Cheng et al., 1995b; Cheng et al., 1993; Cheng et al., 1996b). The second parameter ($D^{0.5}Q^{-0.28}$) was later derived by Cheng et al. (2003) based on *in vivo* nasal deposition data, which exhibited a greater dependence on flow rate (i.e., exponent of -0.28) than the replica-based parameter (i.e., exponent of -0.125). Figures 10a and 10b shows the comparison of deposition profiles for the 53-year-old adult plotted as a function of the above two diffusion parameters. It is noted from Fig. 10a that the deposition results do not fully collapse for different flow rates and particle sizes, suggesting that the replica-based parameter ($D^{0.5}Q^{-0.125}$) does not accurately account for the relative

Ultrafine and Fine Aerosol Deposition in the Nasal Airways of a 9-Month-Old Girl, a 5-Year-Old Boy and a 53-Year-Old Male

45

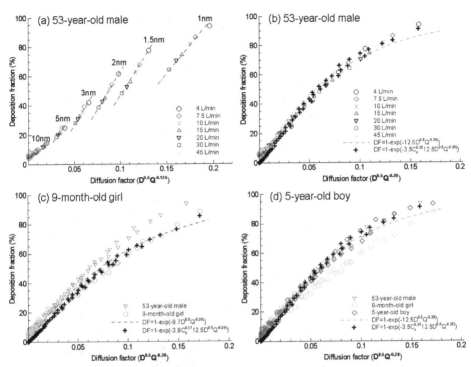

Fig. 10. Comparison of the deposition fractions as a function of the diffusion factor based on existing (a) *in vitro* ($D^{0.5}Q^{-0.125}$) and (b) *in vivo* ($D^{0.5}Q^{-0.28}$) studies in the male adult model. Inclusion of the Cunningham correction factor (C_c) improves agreement between the correlation and numerical data (b). The deposition fractions and associated correlations for (c) 9-month-old girl and (d) 5-year-old boy are also shown as a function of ($D^{0.5}Q^{-0.28}$). Units: Q [L/min] and D [cm²/s].

effect from convection and diffusion. In contrast, a more precise correlation was obtained by plotting the results as a function of the *in-vivo*-based parameter ($D^{0.5}Q^{-0.28}$). Following the format of the *in vivo* empirical correlation suggested by Cheng et al. (2003), $DF = 1 - exp(-a\,D^{0.5}Q^{-0.28})$, a coefficient of $a = 12.5$ was obtained for the 53-year-old deposition results (Fig. 10b). The resulting R^2 value was 0.92, indicating reasonably good agreement between the numerical data and the proposed empirical correlation. However, deviations becomes noticeable from $D^{0.5}Q^{-0.28} = 0.11$ and aggravates thereafter. Considering that deposition in the diffusion regime was also affected by non-continuum effects, the Cunningham correction factor C_c was incorporated into the diffusion parameter as ($C_c^bD^{0.5}Q^{-0.28}$) (Xi and Longest 2009). Again, an equation of $DF = 1 - exp(-c\,C_c^bD^{0.5}Q^{-0.28})$ was used to fit the expiratory simulation data. The best-fit values of b and c were 0.25 and 3.5, respectively, resulting in $R^2 = 0.98$ (Fig. 10b). The resulting ultrafine regime correlation in the nasal-laryngeal airways for adult is expressed as

$$\text{Adult: } DF = 1 - exp(-3.5C_c^{0.25}D^{0.5}Q^{-0.28}) \tag{3}$$

As evident from Fig. 10a and b, inclusion of the Cunningham correction factor results in a better approximation of the numerical data in comparison to the *in-vivo*-based correlation (Fig. 10b), and represents a significant improvement over the replica-based profile in Fig. 10a.

Figures 10c and 10d show the predicted deposition results as a function of $D^{0.5}Q^{-0.28}$ for the 9-month infant and 5-year-old child, respectively. The adult deposition data are also superimposed in these two plots to emphasize the age-related effects. Likewise, better approximations are obtained by including the Cunningham factor for the deposition results of the infant and child, which for the infant is expressed as

$$\text{9-month-old infant: } DF = 1 - \exp(-3.9C_c^{0.17}D^{0.5}Q^{-0.28}) \tag{4}$$

For a given value of diffusion factor ($D^{0.5}Q^{-0.28}$), the deposition results of the infant falls below those of the child and adult, while results of the child and adult appear to collapse into a single curve. As such, the correlation (Eq. 3) is also applied to the 5-year-old child model in this study.

3.5 Sub-regional and local depositions

Sub-regional deposition fractions within specific sections of the nasal airway are illustrated in Figs. 11-13. The sub-regions considered include nasal vestibule and valve (V&V), turbinate region (TR), nasopharynx (NP), pharynx, and larynx, as illustrated in Fig. 2. Figure 11 shows the surface plot of the sub-regional deposition fractions as a function of particle diameter and inhalation flow rate in the 9-month infant model. Surface plots in the child and adult models appear similar and are not shown. Unlike the total deposition plot in Fig. 9a, the flow-deposition response is noted to vary at each sub-region. In the nasopharynx (NP), the deposition fractions appear independent of the flow rate and being a function of particle diameter only (Fig. 11a). Furthermore, in the pharynx region, reduced ultrafine depositions are observed for smaller flow rates, which is opposite to the total deposition plot (Fig. 11 d vs. Fig. 9). This seemingly contrary observation is partially due to the fact that at low flow rates the majority of ultrafine particles entering the nose have deposit in the vestibule and turbinate regions already, leaving only a small amount of particles to deposit in the downstream regions. This depleting mechanism of particles into the anterior nasal passages is more pronounced at even lower inhalation flow rates.

Comparison of sub-regional deposition among the infant, child, and adult models is shown in Fig. 12 for varying particle sizes and in Fig. 13 for varying flow rates. For a same flow rate (15 L/min in Fig. 12), deposition rate consistently decreases with enlarging particles in each sub-region considered. However, this consistency is missing as to the flow rate effect upon the sub-regional deposition for an identical particle size (Fig. 13). Many factors could contribute to the erratic flow-deposition relations in Fig. 13 such as turbulence intensity, secondary motion, particle depletion in upstream regions, etc. In light of age effects, one observation is noteworthy: the deposition partition among the four sub-regions (i.e., turbinate, nasopharynx, pharynx, and larynx) is different for the three airway models. For example, in the turbinate region, the 5-year-old child model receives the highest deposition while the adult model receives the least for all particle sizes and flow rates considered (Figs. 12a, 13a). While in the larynx, the 5-year-old model receives less than the other two models.

Ultrafine and Fine Aerosol Deposition in the Nasal Airways of a 9-Month-Old Girl, a 5-Year-Old Boy and a 53-Year-Old Male

47

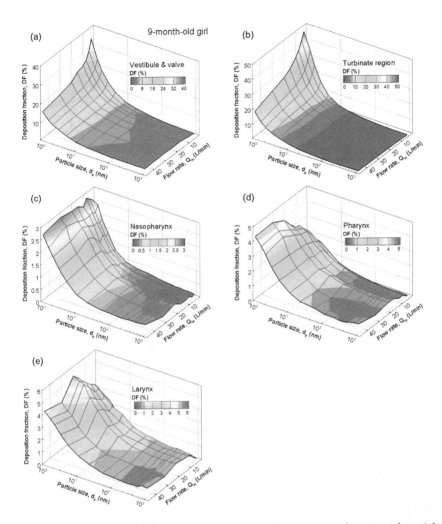

Fig. 11. 3-D surface plot of the sub-regional deposition fractions as a function of particle diameter and inhalation flow rate in the 9-month girl model at the site of (a) nasal vestibule and valve region, (b) turbinate region, (c) nasopharynx, (d) pharynx, and (e) larynx.

Mechanisms behind these irregular partitions could be complex. For example, the nasopharynx in adult has a much larger size and receives a twice larger deposition than in the infant and child. In contrast, the pharynx in child is smallest in size while receives the highest deposition among the three. This finding is worthy of our further attention. For inhalation toxicology, it means a different burden on the region of interest among different age groups. Meanwhile, for inhalation therapy that targets drugs at designated site of the respiratory system, this finding implies that existing adult deposition results might not guarantee an accurate dose planning for children and infants.

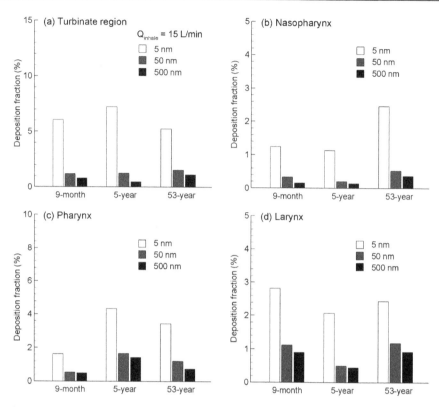

Fig. 12. Comparison of sub-regional deposition fractions between the three models (9-month, 5-year, 53-year) for different particle sizes (5 nm, 50 nm, and 500nm) at the site of (a) turbinate region, (b) nasopharynx, (c) pharynx, and (d) larynx.

To highlight the age-related effects on microdosimetry, a comparison of deposition enhancement factor (DEF) values among the infant, child, and adult models is illustrated in Fig. 14 for particles of 5 nm and an inhalation flow rate of 20 L/min. As discussed, the DEF value quantifies the particle dosage over an area of 50 airway epithelial cells in length with respect to the average deposition rate. The maximum DEF values are of the same order of magnitude for the three subjects considered, i.e. 26 – 41, with the youngest subject having the highest DEF value. This is in contrast with the highly concentrated accumulations of micron aerosols observed in the 5-year-old child model (Xi et al., 2011), which is one order of magnitude higher (i.e., DEF_{max} = 830 for 10 µm particles and 10 L/min flow rate). The overall pattern of deposition enhancement appears very similar for these three models. Each model exhibits hot spots on the dorsal walls of the larynx where convective diffusion is high due to converging airflow to the narrow glottis. Other hot spots with less elevated DEF values are observed for each model in the turbinate region. It is also noted that the nasal valve and pharyngeal dorsal wall do not have significant hot spots, which was the case for 10 µm aerosols (Xi et al., 2011). This lack of hot spots in the valve and pharynx regions is due to the negligible inertial impaction effect for ultrafine particles which can closely follow the main flow and easily maneuver through the constricted or highly curved passages.

Ultrafine and Fine Aerosol Deposition in the Nasal Airways of a 9-Month-Old Girl, a 5-Year-Old Boy and a 53-Year-Old Male

49

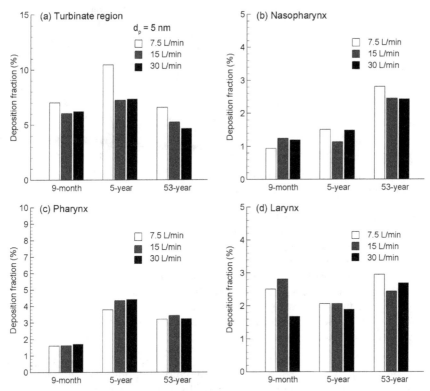

Fig. 13. Comparison of sub-regional deposition fractions between the three models (9-month, 5-year, 53-year) for different inhalation flow rates (7.5 L/min, 15 L/min, and 30 L/min) at the site of (a) turbinate region, (b) nasopharynx, (c) pharynx, and (d) larynx.

Local depositions for nanoparticles of sizes other than 5 nm and for different breathing conditions have been studied but not shown. Generally, it is found that for larger nanoparticles, existing hot spots shrink in size and become more concentrated due to rising particle inertia while deposition in other areas becomes more uniform due to decreased particle diffusivities. For 100 nm aerosols, hot spots reduce to regions only surrounding the glottis. Further, particles are more evenly distributed for heavier activity conditions.

4. Discussion

Significant differences were noted of the nasal anatomy among the infant, child, and adult subjects considered. These differences manifest themselves not only in airway dimension but also in airway morphology. For example, the nasal airway volume of the 9-month-old infant and the 5-year-old child is 18.8% and 40.3% that of the adult, respectively. At the same time, the infant and child have smaller sized nostrils, a shorter turbinate region, and a much slender nasopharynx. Results of this study indicate that the nasal valve and vestibule region might mature around the age of five. This is supported by the much shorter nostril-valve distance (i.e., 11.2 mm for infant *vs.* 20.8 mm for child and 27.2 mm for adult) and

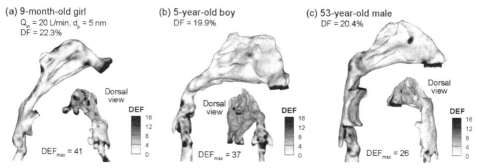

Fig. 14. Comparison of deposition enhancement factors (DEF) at Q_{in} = 20 L/min and d_p = 5 nm in (a) 9-month-old girl, (b) 5-year-old boy, and (c) 53-year-old male.

much smaller valve cross-sectional area (i.e., 56 mm² for infant vs. ~180 mm² for child and adult) of the 9-month infant compared to the 5-year-old child and adult (Fig. 4). The turbinate region experiences fast growth from birth to the age of five as indicated by the remarkable volume increase of this region in Table 2 (i.e., 2.83 cm³ for infant, 11.03 cm³ for child, and 12.63 cm³ for adult); however, a lack of similarity in shape between the child and adult may still mean an undeveloped turbinate. It is apparent that the nasopharynx grows the least during the first five years (i.e., volume = 1.74 cm³ for infant, 3.95 cm³ for child, and 16.33 cm³ for adult, Table 2). These child-adult discrepancies necessitate studies of specific age groups, or of the associated age effects.

Respiratory disorders are diverse in etiology and manifestations. Knowing detailed deposition information will greatly facilitate causality identification and dose-response assessment. The sub-regional and localized deposition values herein, which are amongst the first studies characterizing the detailed depositions in infants and children, have implications in narrowing down or pinpointing the site of highest possibility site (SHP) for respiratory lesions. These deposition hot spots are most susceptible to cancer formation, and are therefore extremely important to identify. For instance, a recent report by the National Research Council (NRC 2008) indicates that the *in vivo* response to inhaled bioaerosols is largely dependent on the site of local particle deposition within the respiratory tract. In this study, the deposition hot spots occur mainly on the turbinate and the dorsal wall of the larynx. Besides, the deposition partition in sub-regions (i.e., turbinate, nasopharynx, pharynx, and larynx) is quite different among the three age groups, indicating a different level of burdens upon the region of interest even when exposed to the same environment. From the drug delivery perspective, this difference finding implies that existing adult deposition results might not guarantee an accurate dose planning for children and infants.

While multiple empirical correlations of nasal nanoparticle depositions exist for adult and to a lesser extent for children, correlations including the age-related effects have rarely been reported. A significant issue in accounting for age effects is to determine the appropriate parameter that best represents the variations of nasal morphology and dimension with age. This parameter could be biological data such as age, height, weight, head circumference, or nasal airway data itself such as volume, surface area, hydraulic diameter, or even a combination of the two. Even though a single correlation applicable to all age groups is highly desirable, such a correlation has to be awaited until more nasal morphology and

Ultrafine and Fine Aerosol Deposition in the Nasal Airways of a 9-Month-Old Girl, a 5-Year-Old Boy and a 53-Year-Old Male

51

deposition data become available for subjects of a large spectrum of ages. It is also a reminder (or caution) that there exist multiple ways in presenting/comparing/extrapolating deposition data in light of the age effects. For instance, besides the ventilation rate as in this study, deposition rates have also been compared in terms of physical activity level (Becquemin et al., 1991), per airway surface area (Diot et al., 1997), and per body mass (Phalen et al., 1991) depending on their comparison purpose. Considering the fact that terminologies defining the ventilation level are relatively arbitrary as no standard definitions exist (Phalen et al., 1985), comparing data from different studies is often not straightforward.

Limitations of this study include the assumptions of steady flow, simplified inlet conditions, ridge airway walls, and non-varying valve and glottal aperture. Other studies have highlighted the physical significance of transient breathing (Shi et al., 2006), inlet velocity profiles (Keyhani et al., 1995; Subramaniam et al., 1998), nasal wall motion (Fodil et al., 2005), nasal valve change (Bridger 1970; Bridger and Proctor 1970) and glottal aperture variation (Brancatisano et al., 1983; Xi et al., 2008). Moreover, each nasal model in this study is based on images of one single subject and does not account for the intersubject variability (Hilberg et al., 1993; Pickering and Beardsmore 1999). Another limitation is the typical supine position of the subjects during data acquisition, which is different from normal breathing while awake. Images are also taken at the end of the inhalation which may not reflect variations in airway geometry during a full breathing cycle. Therefore, future studies are needed that should be orientated toward: (1) improving physical realism and (2) including a broader population group. Our knowledge of nasal deposition is currently lacking in subpopulations such as pediatrics, geriatrics, and patients with respiratory diseases. Due to physiological development, aging, or diseases states, the airway anatomy can be remarkably different from that of a healthy adult. Concentrating on these specific subpopulations will help to clarify inter-group and inter-individual variability and will allow for the design of more efficient pharmaceutical formulations and drug delivery protocols. In particular, future *in vivo* and *in vitro* studies are needed to cross-validate numerical predictions before such results as in this study can be applied to clinical applications.

5. Conclusion

In conclusion, this study has assessed the age-related effects on airflows, breathing impedance, and submicrometer particle depositions in the nasal airways of a 9-month girl, a 5-year-old boy, and a 53-year-old male. A wide spectrum of breathing conditions (3–45 L/min) and aerosol sizes (1–1,000 nm) have been studied by means of numerical simulations. Specific findings of this study include:

1. Significant infant-child-adult discrepancies exist in the nasal airways in both morphology and dimension. Overall, the younger subject has smaller nostrils, a shorter turbinate region, and a slender nasopharynx. Besides, the 9-month infant has much shorter nostril-valve distance and much smaller valve cross-sectional area relative to the 5-year-old child and adult, while those of the later two subjects are similar in size, indicating a maturing of nasal valve at early ages (~ 5 years old). The nasal airway volume of the infant and child is 18.8% and 40.3% that of the adult, respectively; while the nasal airway surface area of the infant and child is 30.0% and 65.7% that of the adult, respectively.

2. Airflow in the main nasal passages was mostly laminar and transitional for all models considered at an inhalation flow rate of 20 L/min, with turbulence occurring mainly in the pharynx and larynx regions.

3. For a same flow rate, breathing resistance persistently decreases with rising age for the three models in this study. An empirical correlation for the breathing resistance was developed for different age groups based on a wide range of test conditions.

4. Insignificant variations in total and local depositions were found among the three models, even though discernible differences can still be noted for hot spot locations and intensities. However, the deposition partitioning in the sub-regions (i.e., turbinate, nasopharynx, pharynx, and larynx) was quite different among the three models considered.

5. Improved correlations of nasal deposition for ultrafine aerosols were developed for different age groups by implementing an *in vivo*-based diffusion parameter and the Cunningham correction factor. These correlations can also be applied to depositions of gases and vapors in the nasal airway for cases of rapid absorption on the airway surface.

6. References

Asgharian, B., Menache, M. G., and Miller, F. J. (2004) Modeling age-related particle deposition in humans. *Journal of Aerosol Medicine*. 17(3), 213-224.

Balashazy, I., Hofmann, W., and Heistracher, T. (1999) Computation of local enhancement factors for the quantification of particle deposition patterns in airway bifurcations. *Journal of Aerosol Science*. 30, 185-203.

Becquemin, M., Swift, D. L., Bouchikhi, A., Roy, M., and Teillac, A. (1991) Particle deposition and resistance in the noses of adults and children. *European Respiratory Journal*. 4(6), 694-702.

Bernstein, G. M. (2004) A review of the influence of particle size, puff volume, and inhalation pattern on the deposition of cigarette smoke particles in the respiratory tract. *Inhalation Toxicology*. 16, 675-689.

Brancatisano, T., Collett, P. W., and Engel, L. A. (1983) Respiratory movements of the vocal cords. *Journal of Applied Physiology*. 54(4), 1269-1276.

Bridger, G. P. (1970) Physiology of nasal valve. *Archives of Otolaryngology*. 92(6), 543-553.

Bridger, G. P., and Proctor, D. F. (1970) Maximum nasal inspiratory flow and nasal resistance. *Annals of Otology Rhinology and Laryngology*. 79(3), 481-488.

California EPA. (2005) *Proposed Identification of Environmental Tobacco Smoke as a Toxic Air Contaminant. Part B: Health Effects*, Sacramento, CA: California Environmental Protection Agency, Office of Environmental Health Hazard Assessment.

Cheng, Y. S., Yamada, Y., Yeh, H. C., and Swift, D. L. (1988) Diffusional deposition of ultrafine aerosols in a human nasal cast. *Journal of Aerosol Science*. 19, 741-751.

Cheng, Y. S., Su, Y. F., Yeh, H. C., and Swift, D. L. (1993) Deposition of Thoron progeny in human head airways. *Aerosol Science and Technology*. 18, 359-375.

Cheng, K.-H., Cheng, Y.-S., Yeh, H.-C., and Swift, D. L. (1995a) Deposition of ultrafine aerosols in the head airways during natural breathing and during simulated breath holding using replicate human upper airway casts. *Aerosol Science and Technology*. 23(3), 465-474.

Ultrafine and Fine Aerosol Deposition in the Nasal Airways of a 9-Month-Old Girl, a 5-Year-Old Boy and
a 53-Year-Old Male

53

Cheng, Y. S., Smith, S. M., Yeh, H. C., Kim, D. B., Cheng, K. H., and Swift, D. L. (1995b) Deposition of ultrafine aerosols and thoron progeny in replicas of nasal airways of young children. *Aerosol Science and Technology*. 23, 541-552.

Cheng, K. H., Cheng, Y. S., Yeh, H. C., Guilmette, R. A., Simpson, S. Q., Yang, S. Q., and Swift, D. L. (1996a) *In vivo* measurements of nasal airway dimensions and ultrafine aerosol depositing in human nasal and oral airways. *Journal of Aerosol Science*. 27, 785-801.

Cheng, Y. S., Yeh, H. C., Guilmette, R. A., Simpson, S. Q., Cheng, K. H., and Swift, D. L. (1996b) Nasal deposition of ultrafine particles in human volunteers and its relationship to airway geometry. *Aerosol Science and Technology*. 25(3), 274-291.

Cheng, Y. S. (2003) Aerosol deposition in the extrathoracic region. *Aerosol Science and Technology*. 37, 659-671.

Cohen Hubal, E. A., Kimbell, J. S., and Fedkiw, P. S. (1996) Incorporation of nasal-lining mass-transfer resistance into a CFD model for prediction of ozone dosimetry in the upper respiratory tract. *Inhalation Toxicology*. 8(9), 831-857.

Crawford, D. J. (1982) Identifying critical human subpopulations by age groups: radioactivity and the lung. *Physics in Medicine and Biology*. 27(4), 539-552.

Diot, P., Palmer, Lucy B., Smaldone, A., Decelie-Germana, J., Grimson, R., and Smaldone, Gerald C. (1997) RhDNase I aerosol deposition and related factors in cystic fibrosis. *American Journal of Respiratory and Critical Care Medicine*. 156(5), 1662-1668.

Eccles, R. (1996) A role for the nasal cycle in respiratory defence. *European Respiratory Journal*. 9(2), 371-376.

Everard, M. L. (2003) Inhalation therapy for infants. *Advanced Drug Delivery Reviews*. 55(7), 869-878.

Fodil, R., Brugel-Ribere, L., Croce, C., Sbirlea-Apiou, G., Larger, C., Papon, J. F., Delclaux, C., Coste, A., Isabey, D., and Louis, B. (2005) Inspiratory flow in the nose: a model coupling flow and vasoerectile tissue distensibility. *Journal of Applied Physiology*. 98(1), 288-295.

Gradon, L., and Yu, C. P. (1989) Diffusional particle depositoin in the human nose and mouth. *Aerosol Science and Technology*. 11, 213-220.

Guilmette, R. A., Cheng, Y. S., Yeh, H. C., and Swift, D. L. (1994) Deposition of 0.005 - 12 micrometer monodisperse particles in a computer-milled, MRI-based nasal airway replica. *Inhalation Toxicology*. 6 (Suppl. 1), 395-399.

Gurr J. R., Wang A. S. S., Chen C. H., Jan K.Y. (2005) Ultrafine titanium dioxide particles in the absence of photoactivation can induce oxidative damage to human bronchial epithelial cells. *Toxicology*, 213, 66-73.

Hilberg, O., Jensen, F. T., and Pedersen, O. F. (1993) Nasal airway geometry: comparison between acoustic reflections and magnetic resonance scanning. *Journal of Applied Physiology*. 75(6), 2811-2819.

ICRP. (1994) *Human Respiratory Tract Model for Radiological Protection*, Elsevier Science Ltd., New York.

Janssens, H. M., de Jongste, J. C., Fokkens, W. J., Robben, S. G., Wouters, K., and Tiddens, H. A. (2001) The Sophia Anatomical Infant Nose-Throat (Saint) model: a valuable tool to study aerosol deposition in infants. *Journal of Aerosol Medicine : The Official Journal of the International Society for Aerosols in Medicine*. 14(4), 433-41.

Keith, C. H. (1982) Particle size studies on tobacco smoke. *Beiträge zur Tabakforschung International/Contributions to Tobacco Research.* 11(3), 123-131.

Kelly, J. T., Asgharian, B., Kimbell, J. S., and Wong, B. (2004a) Particle deposition in human nasal airway replicas manufactured by different methods. Part I: inertial regime particles. *Aerosol Science and Technology.* 38, 1063-1071.

Kelly, J. T., Asgharian, B., Kimbell, J. S., and Wong, B. (2004b) Particle deposition in human nasal airway replicas manufactured by different methods. Part II: ultrafine particles. *Aerosol Science and Technology.* 38, 1072-1079.

Keyhani, K., Scherer, P. W., and Mozell, M. M. (1995) Numerical simulation of airflow in the human nasal cavity. *Journal of Biomechanical Engineering-Transactions of the Asme.* 117(4), 429-441.

Kittelson, D. B. (1998) Engines and nanoparticles: a review. *Journal of Aerosol Science.* 29(5-6), 575-588.

Kreyling, W. G., Semmler-Behnke, M., and Moller, W. (2006) Ultrafine particle-lung interactions: does size matter? *Journal of Aerosol Medicine.* 19, 74-83.

Kreyling, W. G., Semmler, M., and Moller, W. (2004) Dosimetry and toxicology of ultrafine particles. *Journal of Aerosol Medicine.* 17(2), 140-152.

Li, N., Sioutas, C., Cho, A., Schmitz, D., Misra, C., Sempf, J., Wang, M. Y., Oberley, T., Froines, J., and Nel, A. (2003) Ultrafine particulate pollutants induce oxidative stress and mitochondrial damage. *Environmental Health Perspectives.* 111(4), 455-460.

Liu, Y., Matida, E. A., Gu, J., and Johnson, M. R. (2007) Numerical simulation of aerosol deposition in a 3-D human nasal cavity using RANS, RANS/EIM, and LES. *Journal of Aerosol Science.* 38, 683-700.

Longest, P. W., and Xi, J. (2007) Effectiveness of direct Lagrangian tracking models for simulating nanoparticle deposition in the upper airways. *Aerosol Science and Technology.* 41, 380-397.

Lumb, A. B. (2000) *Nunn's Applied Respiratory Physiology,* Butterworth Heinemann, Oxford.

Mandell, G. L., Bennett, J. E., and Bolin, R. D. (2004) *Principles and Practices of Infectious Diseases,* Churchhill Livingstone, New York.

Martonen, T. B. (1986) Surrogate experimental models for studying particle deposition in the human respiratory tract: an overview. *Aerosols,* S. D. Lee, ed., Lewis Publishers, Chesea, Michigan.

Martonen, T. B., Zhang, Z. Q., Yue, G., and Musante, C. J. (2003) Fine particle deposition within human nasal airways. *Inhalation Toxicology.* 15(4), 283-303.

Matida, E. A., Finlay, W. H., Lang, C. F., and Grgic, L. B. (2004) Improved numerical simulation of aerosol deposition in an idealized mouth-throat. *Journal of Aerosol Science.* 35, 1-19.

Morsi, S. A., and Alexander, A. J. (1972) An investigation of particle trajectories in two-phase flow systems. *Journal of Fluid Mechanics.* 55(2), 193-208.

NRC. (2008) *A Framework for Assessing teh Health Hazad Posed by Bioaerosols,* The national Academies Press, Washington DC.

Oberdorster, G., and Utell, M. J. (2002) Ultrafine particles in the urban air: to the respiratory tract and beyond. *Environmental Health Perspectives.* 110(8), A440-A441.

Oldham, M. J., Mannix, R. C., and Phalen, R. F. (1997) Deposition of monodisperse particles in hollow models representing adult and child-size tracheobroncial airways. *Health Physics.* 72(6), 827-833.

Ultrafine and Fine Aerosol Deposition in the Nasal Airways of a 9-Month-Old Girl, a 5-Year-Old Boy and
a 53-Year-Old Male

55

Ostiguy, C., Soucy, B., Lapointe G., Woods. C., Menard, L., and Trottier M., (2008) Health effects of nanoparticles, seond edition, in *Chemical Substance and Biological Agents*, Report R-589, IRSST, Montreal.

Phalen, R. F., Cuddihy, R. G., Fisher, R. G., Moss, O. R., Schlesinger, R. B., Swift, D. L., and Yeh, H. C. (1991) Main features of the proposed NCRP respiratory tract dosimetry model. *Radiation Protection Dosimetry*. 38, 179-184.

Phalen, R. F., Oldham, M. J., Beaucage, C. B., Crocker, T. T., and Mortensen, J. D. (1985) Postnatal enlargement of human tracheobronchial airways and implications for particle deposition. *The Anatomical Record*. 212, 368-380.

Pickering, D. N., and Beardsmore, C. S. (1999) Nasal flow limitation in children. *Pediatric Pulmonology*. 27(1), 32-36.

Pritchard, S. E., and McRobbie, D. W. (2004) Studies of the human oropharyngeal airspaces using magnetic resonance imaging. II. The use of three-dimensional gated MRI to determine the influence of mouthpiece diameter and resistance of inhalation devices on the oropharyngeal airspace geometry. *Journal of Aerosol Medicine*. 17(4), 310-324.

Sayes, C. M., Gobin, A. M., Ausman, K. D., Mendez. J., West, J. L., Colvin, V. L. (2005) Nano-C60 cytotoxicity is due to lipid peroxidation. *Biomaterials*, 25, 7587-7595.

Scherer, P. W., Keyhani, K., and Mozell, M. M. (1994) Nasal dosimetry modeling for humans. *Inhalation Toxicology*. 6, 85-97.

Schroeter, J. D., Musante, C. J., Hwang, D. M., Burton, R., Guilmette, R., and Martonen, T. B. (2001) Hygroscopic growth and deposition of inhaled secondary cigarette smoke in human nasal pathways. *Aerosol Science and Technology*. 34(1), 137-143.

Shi, H., Kleinstreuer, C., and Zhang, Z. (2006) Laminar airflow and nanoparticle or vapor deposition in a human nasal cavity model. *Journal of Biomechanical Engineering*. 128, 697-706.

Subramaniam, R. P., Richardson, R. B., Morgan, K. T., Kimbell, J. S., and Guilmette, R. A. (1998) Computational fluid dynamics simulations of inspiratory airflow in the human nose and nasopharynx. *Inhalation Toxicology*. 10(2), 91-120.

Swift, D. L., and Strong, J. C. (1996) Nasal deposition of ultrafine 218Po aerosols in human subjects. *Journal of Aerosol Science*. 27(7), 1125-1132.

U.S. Surgeon General Report. (2007) *Children and Secondhand Smoke Exposure-Excerpts from The Health Consequences of Involuntary Exposure to Tobacco Smoke: A Report of the Surgeon General*, U.S. Department of Health and Human Services.

Wheatley, J. R., Amis, T. C., and Engel, L. A. (1991) Nasal and oral airway pressure-flow relationships. *Journal of Applied Physiology*. 71(6), 2317-2324.

Wilcox, D. C. (1998) *Turbulence Modeling for CFD, 2nd Ed.*, DCW Industries, Inc., California.

Xi, J., and Longest, P. W. (2007) Transport and deposition of micro-aerosols in realistic and simplified models of the oral airway. *Annals of Biomedical Engineering*. 35(4), 560-581.

Xi, J., and Longest, P. W. (2008) Numerical predictions of submicrometer aerosol deposition in the nasal cavity using a novel drift flux approach. *International Journal of Heat and Mass Transfer*. 51(23-24), 5562-5577.

Xi, J., Longest, P. W., and Martonen, T. B. (2008) Effects of the laryngeal jet on nano- and microparticle transport and deposition in an approximate model of the upper tracheobronchial airways. *Journal of Applied Physiology*. 104(6), 1761-1777.

Xi, J., and Longest, P. W. (2009) Characterization of submicrometer aerosol deposition in extrathoracic airways during nasal exhalation. *Aerosol Science and Technology.* 43(8), 808-827.

Xi, J., Longest, P. W., and Anderson P. J. (2010) Respiratory aerosol dyanmics with applications to pharmaceutical drug delivery, in *Colloids in Drug Delivery,* Monzer Fanun (ed.), CRC Press Taylor & Francis, 501-526.

Xi, J., Si, X., Kim, J. W., and Berlinski, A. (2011) Simulation of airflow and aerosol deposition in the nasal cavity of a 5-year-old child. *Journal of Aerosol Science.* 42(3), 156-173.

Xu, G. B., and Yu, C. P. (1986) Effects of Age on Deposition of Inhaled Aerosols in the Human Lung. *Aerosol Science and Technology.* 5(3), 349-357.

Yamada, Y., Cheng, Y. S., Yeh, H. C., and Swift, D. L. (1988) Inspiratory and expiratory deposition of ultrafine particles in a human nasal cast. *Inhalation Toxicology.* 1, 1-11.

Yang, C. P., Callagher, R. P., Weiss, N. S., B and, P. R., Thomas, D. B., and Russel, D. A. (1989) Differences in incidence rates of cancers of the respiratory tract by anatomic subside and histological type: an etiologic implication. *Journal of National Cancer Institute.* 81(21), 1828-1831.

Yu, G., Zhang, Z., and Lessmann, R. (1998) Fluid flow and particle diffusion in the human upper respiratory system. *Aerosol Science and Technology.* 28, 146.

Zamankhan, P., Ahmadi, G., Wang, Z., Hopke, P. K., Cheng, Y. S., Su, W. C., and Leonard, D. (2006) Airflow and deposition of nano-particles in a human nasal cavity. *Aerosol Science and Technology.* 40, 463-476.

Zhao, K., Scherer, P. W., Hajiloo, S. A., and Dalton, P. (2004) Effects of anatomy on human nasal air flow and odorant transport patterns: implications for olfaction. *Chemical Senses.* 29(5), 365-379.

4

Safety, Security and Quality: Lessons from GMO Risk Assessments

Alice Benessia[1,2] and Giuseppe Barbiero[1,3]
[1]*Interdisciplinary Research Institute on Sustainability*
[2]*Università degli studi di Torino*
[3]*Università della Valle d'Aosta*
Italy

1. Introduction

Assessing the impact of new techno-sciences on our life supporting systems and on our present and future common wealth is a complex and controversial issue that involves the relation between science and governance, and more generally, between science and democracy (Gallopin *et al.*, 2001).

Indeed, governments find themselves in the contradictory role of *speeding up* techno-scientific innovation, in order to maintain market share and hence economic survival in the globalized competition system, and of *slowing down* the very same process, in order to keep ensuring one of the main pillars of modern states: safety. Concurrently, as we will see, scientific research carries out the equivalent conflicting task of producing knowledge for innovation *and* for regulation. Finally, citizens demand safety, but the very reassuring certainty they require, paradoxically undermines the confidence they hold in the capacity of modern state to ensure this fundamental right; indeed, admitting a danger seems more trust worthy than declaring the absence of risks, especially after major crises in the regulatory system, such as the one of bovine spongiform encephalopathy (BSE). In these epistemic and normative tensions - defined as a "Triple Catch 23" by the British philosopher Jerome Ravetz (Ravetz, 2003) - new relationships between science, society and governance need to be investigated and implemented (De Marchi & Ravetz, 1999).

As we will articulate, the modern ideal of grounding our decision-making processes on the certain, objective and exhaustive knowledge, produced by an independent community of scientists - in other words the principle of 'science speaking truth to power'- is inadequate when applied to our contemporary open-field, irreversible experimentation, characterized by intrinsic complexity and controversy.

Complexity entails the paradoxical epistemic situation according to which the more we know about the interaction between social and environmental systems and the more there is to know. Lack of certainty, namely uncertainty and ignorance, is therefore not temporary or accidental, but intrinsic and unavoidable. On the other hand, *controversy* implies the inherent and inextricable coupling between facts and values, and therefore the existence of mutually incompatible and indispensable epistemic and normative perspectives. Under these conditions, typically 'post-normal' (Funtowicz & Ravetz, 1993) a certain, objective and exhaustive knowledge for a rational decision can never be achieved nor even conceived of.

In this chapter, we would like to propose some critical reflections on the underlying assumptions and consequences of the conception and use of risk assessment techniques, by contextualizing them to this broader scenario.

As exemplary cases, we will focus our attention on the role and impact of biotechnologies on the global food production systems. More specifically, we will proceed by reviewing and analyzing, in this more extensive epistemic and normative context, different open questions about the impact of genetically modified organisms in agriculture (Guarnieri *et al.*, 2008) and in aquaculture (Barbiero *et al.*, 2011).

We will first start from clarifying the main critical aspects inherent in defining and assessing the risks of these techno-scientific processes and products. Complexity and controversy will be explored in terms of the unavoidable presence of ignorance, the coexistence of multiple disciplinary perspectives and epistemic cultures, and the aims and stakes dependency of any framing of risk.

Innovation, precautionary and regulatory science, namely the three modes of scientific research involved in the production, impact evaluation and regulation of biotechnology will be then defined and examined, in relation to their corresponding epistemic and normative cultures and *praxis*. The driving argument will be to show that both production and regulation are driven by the epistemic culture of innovation, based on the principles of certainty, objectivity and exhaustiveness, and enclosed in a modern, evidence-based epistemic and normative black box. We will also argue that three grand narratives of innovation, founded on the ideals of control, power and urgency, are in charge of normalizing whatever comes from out of the box, i.e. complexity and controversy.

In this scenario, by focusing on the so called negative and liminal knowledge (Kastenhofer, 2010, Knorr Cetina, K. 1999), the key role of *precautionary science* is to peak in, and ultimately to break in the box of the whole innovation and regulation process (Jasanoff, 2005), leaving room for a democratized, open and post-normal evaluation of bio-technologies.

A first step in shading some light through the actual complexity involved in the genetic engineering endeavor will be to examine the crisis of the central dogma of molecular biology, as emerged from the past two decades of research. The founding pillars of the biotech production system - determinism, reductionism and mechanism - are indeed facing a deep challenge, given the numerous evidence of the actual complexity of the genome's physiology. When fully acknowledged the repercussions of this crisis could destabilize the entire edifice of *biotech* industry, including the normative foundations of genetic engineering's patenting law.

We will then deepen and extend our reflection on the impacts of Genetically Modified Organisms (GMOs) by analyzing some of the main controversies involved in the open-field agri-food implementation, correlating them with the notions of food (bio)safety, security and quality.

(Bio)safety is traditionally associated with the absence of possible environmental and health hazards, and therefore correlated to and defined *by* risk assessments[1]. We will explore this correlation and its relations with the grand narrative of control.

We will then move to the global issue of food security, commonly referred to as the availability of and the stable access to healthy food supplies. In this respect, we will examine the grand narrative of power according to which (only) biotechnology enhanced crops and animals can and will feed our overpopulated world. As we will see, on the one hand GMOs are evaluated and regulated in terms of their *safety*, on the other hand they are promoted in terms of their necessity for achieving food *security*. The latter argument is improperly utilized to reinforce the former, according to the third grand narrative of innovation, namely urgency. In this view, GMOs can and should be considered *safe enough*, given their role in tackling present and future global hunger. Indeed, both the possible correlation between safety and security and the actual need for GMOs in dealing with food security are highly controversial (Altieri & Rosset, 1999; Francescon, 2006; Giampietro, 2009; Waltner-Toews & Lang, 2000).

Finally, we will step into the necessity of moving from safety and security to the issue of food *quality* in its crucial connection with the development and use of new *narratives of humility* (Jasanoff, 2003), grounded on a thoughtful diagnosis of the *present* distribution of techno-scientific, cultural, economic and political power and of local and global vulnerability to change (Funtowicz & Strand, 2011).

This analysis will lead us to outline a number of paradoxes embodied in the conception and use of risk assessment techniques. The traditional western reaction to paradoxes is to try to solve them, but we believe that another fruitful approach, typical of other cultural traditions and revitalized in the post-normal scenario (Ravetz, 2001), can be useful in this case: to accept the paradoxes and to constructively and creatively learn from them about the limitations of our own existing intellectual structures.

2. Deciding under lack of knowledge: From experiment to experience

2.1 High-power open-field experimentation: Complexity, irreversibility and controversy

Over the last century, the intensity, the time scale and the diffusion of our technological intervention on natural, cultural and social systems have grown exponentially. We are now able to act on socio-ecological systems with an unprecedented power. In a more literal sense, we are manipulating matter and energy over shorter and shorter time frames, interfering locally and globally with the bio-geo-chemical cycles of our planet (Elser & Bennet, 2011; Rockström *et al.*, 2009; Townsend & Howarth, 2010).

At the same time, the boundaries of disciplinary science and technological enterprises and profits have been steadily blurring, with the oligopolization of industrial production systems. Corporate know-how has been gradually expanding at the expense of common

---

[1] We will utilize the synthesizing term of (bio)safety to refer to both health and environmental risks, focusing our specific attention on the latter, but keeping in mind the existence of equivalent debate about the former.

knowledge. From the epistemic and normative closure of our simplified, controlled and reversible scientific laboratory practice, we have been stepping into a variety of open-field techno-scientific direct experimentations.

This overall transition entails at least three kinds of consequences (Benessia, 2009). First, the interaction between socio-ecological systems and technology itself is characterized by emergent and reflexive complexity (Funtowicz & Ravetz, 1994). Radically different from the mere simplifiable complication of laboratory settings, emergent complexity implies tight coupling between different levels of organization, interacting and influencing each other through highly non-linear dynamics, critical dependence from initial conditions, and self-organizing emergent properties. Concurrently, the presence in the socio-environmental systems of elements provided with individuality, intentionality, autonomous aims, foresight, symbolic representations and morality entails a level of reflexive complexity. Knowledge about the evolution of complex systems is therefore always incomplete and surprise is inevitable (Gallopin, 2001). In this situation, our ability to predict the outcomes of our actions is radically undermined by the quality and the magnitude of what we do not and cannot possibly know. Indeed, when dealing with emergent and reflexive complexity, the kind of knowledge we lack is intrinsically different from quantifiable risk: uncertainty, ignorance and indeterminacy dominate our cognitive endeavours about future developments. Following Smith and Wynne's (1989) classification of the lack of knowledge relating to different decision-making modalities, one speaks of risk when the main variables of the problem are known and the respective probabilities of different outcomes are quantifiable and quantified. A typical example is the risk of losing when playing roulette, characterized by a known, closed, finite and discreet information space. Uncertainty is associated with a situation in which the main variables of the problem are known, but the quantitative incidence of the relevant factors is not and it is therefore impossible to assign different probabilities to different events. It can also be defined as a probability of second order, in which different risks assessment scenarios associated with different distributions of probability are compared (Bodansky, 1994; Tallacchini, 2005). Lack of knowledge is defined as ignorance when even the main variables of the problem are unknown and therefore the probabilities of negative outcomes are also unknown. Ignorance is unavoidable when dealing with evolving systems, in which the information space is open and expanding (Giampietro, 2002; Prigogine, 1978). Finally, as we will further explore, indeterminacy is correlated with the presence of multiple and non-reducible epistemic and normative perspectives (Sarewitz, 2004).

The second relevant consequence of our contemporary high-power techno-scientific implementation is that direct open-field experimentation is by definition irreversible. If something goes wrong we cannot run a second test. This mere fact implies that, unlike what happens in the laboratory practice, we cannot proceed by iterative approximations to the result we want, avoiding on the way what we do not want. In other words, just like with life experiences, we don't have the luxury of painlessly learning from our mistakes.

When considered together, these two consequences amount to the possibility of unforeseen, unpredictable and unrecoverable negative outcomes. Contemporary techno-science is then supposed to deliver ever-new 'goods', but it is also concurrently exposing socio-environmental systems to ever-new possible corresponding 'bads'. In his prescient book on "normal accidents", Charles Perrow reflects on the inexorable occurrence of harmful events

– accidents – as a consequence of the reflexive complexity and the tight coupling inherent in our high-power technologies (Perrow, 1984). A few years later, in defining our contemporary techno-scientifically driven way of life as "risk society", Ulrich Beck refers to this controversial condition of modernization, in which risks are woven into the very fabric of progress (Beck, 1986).

Finally, whereas the supposed benefits of techno-scientific processes and products are 'built in' within industrially optimized and controlled systems, their possible serious drawbacks cannot be addressed by a single scientific discipline and framework, or more generally by techno-science alone. These problematic circumstances, which were effectively captured by Alvin Weinberg's as "transcientific" in the early seventies (Weinberg, 1972), lead us to the third fundamental consequence of open-field, high-power experimentation: the absence of a predefined scientific disciplinary framing, setting and method of inquiry, in foreseeing and managing the effects of techno-scientific implementation over the systems involved. Multiple and incommensurable perspectives, such as modes of questioning, detecting, measuring, even identifying relevant data, are meant to coexist indefinitely precisely because the objects of inquiry do not emerge from a predetermined laboratory and disciplinary set up. This plurality of relevant, indispensable and often incompatible standpoints determines a level of indeterminacy (Smith & Wynne, 1989) in the very definition of the issues at stake. Moreover, as we will further explore, different epistemologies, ontologies and methodologies involve as many normative stances. In Daniel Sarewitz's words: "The necessity of looking at nature through a variety of disciplinary lenses brings with it a variety of normative lenses, as well" (Sarewitz, 2004). In this inherent and inextricable coupling between facts and values, which we will refer to as controversy, negotiation and most often competition between disciplines - and their related normative power - becomes a founding criterion for choosing what kind of knowledge is "scientifically relevant" for the issue at stake.

In this overall scenario, if we cannot accurately predict, exhaustively describe, and effectively remove the consequences of our action, then a deep reflection on the grounds and methodologies of what we call responsible decision and conduct is needed.

2.2 From the modern model to post-normal science

When complex socio-environmental systems are involved, the modern ideal of founding our decision-making processes on the neutral knowledge produced by an independent community of scientists – in other words of 'scientists speaking truth to power' (Wildavsky, 1979) - becomes inadequate. Complexity, irreversibility and indeterminacy radically undermine the idea that science can provide a single, certain, objective and exhaustive perspective from which a straightforward decision can be taken at a political level.

A first acknowledgement of this kind of procedural inadequacy was internationally made in 1992, in the Principle 15 of Rio Declaration on Environment and Development, in which a precautionary approach was invoked: "In order to protect the environment the precautionary approach shall be widely applied by States according to their capabilities. Where there are threats of serious and irreversible damage, lack of full scientific certainty shall not be used as a reason for postponing cost-effective measures to prevent environment degradation".

The precautionary approach introduces the idea that science can be temporarily unable to produce a certain and exhaustive body of knowledge suitable for a rational decision. A political stance has then to be introduced in order to minimize the chance of harming people and the environment, over the chance of an economic loss, due to a technological restriction. The fundamental consequence of this normative step is an epistemic shift from a two values theoretical science, based on the evaluation of the truth/falsity of a hypothesis, to a three value science 'applied to risks', which includes uncertainty as a possible outcome of a scientific assessment. This in turn implies a deep change in the modern relationship between scientific truth and the correspondingly right political decision, by introducing the notion of risk acceptability through a normative action (Shrader-Frechette, 1996; Tallacchini, 2005). Indeed, in the 2000 Communication from the European Commission, the precautionary principle is qualified as a principle of political responsibility, namely a principle that considers certain risks as "inconsistent with the high level of protection chosen for the Community" (Communication from the European Commission, 2000).

The precautionary model represents a substantial improvement over the inherent positivism of the modern ideal, in that uncertainty and the need for an eminently political choice are explicitly taken into account. Nonetheless, the privileged nature of scientific knowledge is not challenged at its roots: lack of full knowledge is still regarded as technical uncertainty, a provisional condition ascribable to temporary methodological difficulties in collecting and managing data.

In the same Communication from the European Commission, the precautionary principle is associated with risk management: it can be invoked only when a scientific assessment provides evidence of risk and when the precautionary measures are in line with a proportionality principle between cost and benefits (Funtowicz, 2007). In other words, in this model, lack of knowledge is recognized but improperly reduced to a temporary and statistically manageable condition. Therefore, the presence and the epistemic and normative consequences of emergent complexity, namely ignorance, indeterminacy and controversy, are not fully acknowledged.

In 1993 , around the same time as the Rio Declaration, Silvio Funtowicz and Jerome Ravetz developed a radically new way of conceiving the relationship between science and policy, deeply challenging the modern ideal of the autonomous and privileged 'republic of science' providing 'the facts' to policy makers (Merton, 1968). In this framework (Figure 1), defined as post-normal science, the complexity, irreversibility and indeterminacy involved in contemporary socio-environmental issues are fully acknowledged in all their consequences (Funtowicz & Ravetz, 1993).

The starting point of their reflection is that in the majority of cases in which techno-science is called into question by the normative sphere, facts are uncertain, values are in dispute, decisions are urgent and stakes are high. From the one-dimensional incremental ideal of progress towards certainty, typical of the modern model and of its precautionary development, here we step into a two dimensional representation space, where uncertainty is correlated with decision stakes. This correlation allows discriminating between three fundamentally different kinds of scientific research. In the scenario that we have so far outlined, the transition from one area to the next is determined by incrementing techno-scientific power and therefore the complexity involved.

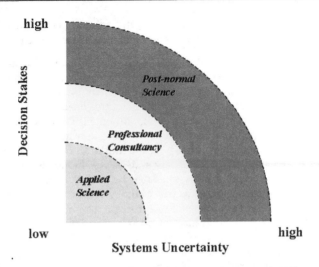

Fig. 1. The framework of post-normal science (Funtowicz & Ravetz, 1993)

The first type of research is *applied science*, essentially laboratory science, in which risks are predictable and under control. The information space is closed and knowable and reductionist approaches can be useful. It is the condition in which the modern model has emerged and it has been easily applied.

When complexity grows and both decision stakes and uncertainty increase, we get into the area of *professional consultancy*, where specifically selected experts advice is required to inform policy makers in order to orient the decision in the most rational and responsible way. As we will later specify, regulatory science and the attempts to extend the modern ideal by protecting scientific knowledge from uncertainty, indeterminacy and abuse can be ascribed to this area (Funtowicz, 2006). In particular, the precautionary approach and the related risk assessment and cost benefits analyses are invoked in this context.

Extending further techno-scientific power, we get into the post-normal science scenario, characterized by the paradoxical situation in which knowing more entails new levels of complexity and therefore more uncertainty, indeterminacy and ignorance. This dynamic implies the necessity of developing new methods of knowledge production and new criteria for assessing their quality (Funtowicz & Ravetz, 1990).

In the modern model of applied science, relevant knowledge is scientific by definition and the quality of scientific knowledge is identified with its degree of "truth", which is autonomously evaluated within the scientific community itself, through the peer review procedure. The implicit assumption is that the normative sphere can and has to be kept apart from the quality assessment process.

In the precautionary approach, typical of professional consultancy, relevant knowledge is still scientific and the quality assessment procedures based on peer review are integrated with new ways to evaluate the degree of acceptability of risk. Despite this wider set of criteria, the separability and the need to preserve the ideal modern separation between the description of the relevant facts, provided by science, and the values of politics is still firmly reconfirmed. In this sense the actual application of the precautionary principle is reduced to a technical fix based on scientific *consensus* rather than truth (Sarewitz, 2011).

But in the context of complex and controversial socio-environmental issues, as expressed in the post-normal model, facts and values are not separable and therefore no form of knowledge, including a scientific one, can be evaluated on the basis of a univocally predefined concept of truth. New forms of public control of knowledge production have then to be elaborated (Funtowicz & Ravetz, 1990). This entails the necessity, not only ethical or political, but primarily epistemic and methodological, to extend the public participation in the decision making processes. From the logical demonstration of evidence-based matter-of-fact, validated by a disciplinary peer review system, we should step into open dialogues including extended facts and collectively validated by extended peer review processes. In this new context: "Science is considered as part of the relevant knowledge and it is included as a part of the probative evidence of a process. The ideal of rigorous scientific demonstration is thus replaced by an ideal of open public dialogue. Inside the knowledge production process, citizens become both critics and creators. Their contribution has not to be defined as 'local', 'practical', 'ethical' or 'spiritual' knowledge, but it has to be considered and accepted as a plurality of rightful and coordinated perspectives with their own meaning and value structures" (Liberatore & Funtowicz, 2003, p. 147, as cited by Tallacchini, 2005).

2.3 Biotechnology for food production: An open debate

In light of what we have outlined so far, let's now turn our attention to one of the most intense and pervasive open-field experimentation of the last few decades: biotechnology for food production. The debate about the impact of this kind of techno-scientific innovation on our socio-ecological systems, over local and global scale, is indeed highly complex and controversial. Moreover, as we will be exploring in the following, it is still rooted in the modern model of interaction between science and policy, despite the numerous attempts to democratize the debate about its consequences.

We will start our investigation on the impact of GMO's in the agri-food system by embedding this issue in the larger context of the dominant epistemic and normative strategies used for assessing and managing the complexity and controversy involved. As we will see, these strategies are essentially founded on a black boxing mechanism, defended through a set of standardizing strategies and narratives of modernity, whereas post-normal approaches are mostly needed but far from being widespread.

3. Biotechnologies in context

3.1 Modes of research and epistemic cultures

As any other techno-scientific endeavour, food related biotechnology depends on science in (at least) three ways: for its production, impact evaluation and regulation.

These three distinct phases, which are all equally crucial, correspond to three distinct modes of scientific research: innovation science, precautionary science and regulatory science. These types of research define and are embedded in a variety of corresponding epistemic cultures (Kastenhofer, 2010), interlinked with a range of disciplinary frameworks and implying distinct normative assumptions, such as evidence framing and detection, focus of interest, quality assurance methodologies and most of all uncertainty management.

Innovation science (Wynne quoted by Jasanoff, 2005) is typically carried out by private industries, not rarely granted with public funds (Goldenberg, 2011), with the explicit aim of developing and introducing new (bio)technological products in the market. The prevalent goal of this type of endeavour is to make things work. This, in turn, entails a methodology founded on laboratory trial-and-error iterative approximation to the desired result, through the design and management of linear cause-effect relationships between a limited or limitable number of variables (i.e. a specific gene for a specific property, according the central dogma ideal which we will discuss in the following section). The corresponding epistemic culture of innovation science is therefore essentially based on determinism, reductionism and mechanism, applied *in vitro*, to small and de-contextualized temporal and spatial horizons, and resulting in the production of so-called hard facts, namely new goods, characterized by a given set of properties, with the externalization of uncertainty.

In the scheme of post-normal science, this kind of epistemic approach evokes the first quadrant, what we referred to as applied science. The main *caveat* to be kept in mind at this point is that, in the case of biotechnology, just as in any other techno-scientific global and direct experimentation, we are not in the modern scenario of laboratory science, as the result of experimenting over living systems in all their intrinsic emergent complexity, and because these products are meant to be diffused and tested directly into open socio-ecological systems. Molecular biology and genetic engineering are the leading disciplines of this type of research.

Precautionary science (Ravetz, 2004) is normally undertaken within research institutions such as universities, and it involves the understanding and the management of the consequences of large-scale techno-scientific implementation. Its main focus is therefore the complexity of interaction between the organisms involved - this time conceived and treated as processes- and the environment. The correlated epistemic culture of this type of scientific research is based on observation *in situ*, through systemic approaches over large population systems and extended temporal and spatial horizons, involving highly non-linear causal links, such as retroaction mechanisms, dependence on initial conditions etc.

Precautionary science also involves an experience-oriented epistemic culture, with middle range temporal and spatial horizons, observation, communication and intervention, strong reliance on individual case history and professional rather than scientific identity (Kastenhofer, 2007)

The disciplinary set up of this mode of research includes ecology, epidemiology, toxicology, plant breeding science, system and population biology.

Whereas innovation science mainly concentrates on producing consistent - and profitable - objects in a controlled way, precautionary science is interested in the so-called negative or liminal knowledge (Kastenhofer, 2010; Knorr Cetina, 1999), implying the extremely ambitious task of investigating the absence of specific – or even unspecified - object characteristics, namely unwanted and harmful properties, the absence of causal relations and the absence of natural processes and mechanisms including such causal relations. Therefore, this kind of epistemic endeavor entails the recognition of complexity and ignorance, and the attempt to manage indeterminacy and irreversibility. As we will see, the main problem with the liminal knowledge of precautionary science is its impractical relation with decision-making processes, still based on the modern model, which requires incontrovertible evidence and hard facts.

This evidence-based ideal is actively pursued by regulatory science (Jasanoff, 1990), within public agencies such as the Food and Drug Administration, by endorsing the innovation science epistemic approach, in most cases even with the aid of the very same people, through the so-called "revolving door" phenomenon between regulatory agencies and industry (Mattera, 2004; Meghani & Kuzma, 2011; Revolving Door Working Group [RDWG], 2005). Leaving aside the most basic issue of conflict of interests and biased epistemic and normative positions, the main critical issue is that regulatory science is characterized by an intrinsic ambivalent position towards uncertainty. On the one hand, just like precautionary science, its aim is to deal with the possible impacts of technological implementation, therefore openly assuming a given lack of knowledge. On the other hand, in order to be credible in the modern scenario, it has to deliver by default a certain, objective and exhaustive factual position towards the issue at stake.

As a result of this tension, the main strategy of regulatory science is to ask only scientifically answerable questions, and then to equate a narrowly defined risk assessment with scientific assessment. The European's implementation of the Precautionary Principle in terms of risks/costs/benefits analyses goes precisely in this direction. This black-boxing epistemic and normative procedure to externalize complexity, indeterminacy and controversy evokes the so-called lamppost paradox, where one searches for the lost keys, at night, only under the lamppost just because it is the only place where one can see (Funtowicz & Strand, 2011). Thus, from the laboratory closure of innovation science, here we step into a form of institutional closure, with the aid of authoritative expert advice, the professional consultancy in the post-normal diagram, belonging to the epistemic culture and – at least in the US - to the actual community of the biotech industrial system.

3.2 The normative implications of regulatory processes and risk assessments

A number of authors have analyzed in details the nature and the implications of this lack of openness. In a seminal work on risks and regulatory processes, Sheila Jasanoff refers to the risks assessment procedures in regulatory frameworks as "technologies of hybris" for three reasons (Jasanoff, 2003, 2007). First, they focus on the known at the expenses of the unknown, on short-term quantitatively manageable risks, leaving in the shadow long-term indeterminate and possibly ignored consequences - the so-called unknown unknowns (European Environmental Agency, 2001).

Second, their capacity to internalize challenges that come from outside their framing assumptions is limited, as in the case of chemical toxicity assessments that continue to rest on "the demonstrably faulty assumption that people are exposed to one chemical at a time" (Jasanoff, 2003: 239).

Third, the specialized language and knowledge used to elaborate and to make use of these technologies in the context of policy tend to preempt an open discussion with all legitimate stakeholders. More specifically, the normative assumptions of these analytic models are not subject to general debate and the modern ideal of objectivity is used as a tool to obscure the boundary work that is needed to design them.

Indeed, a starting point for a deeper reflection on the foundations, functions and aims of regulatory risks assessments is the recognition that they are not and cannot be value-neutral, as they inherently depend on normative assumptions in a variety of ways (Kuzma & Besley

2008; Lewenstein, 2005; Meghani, 2009): in the formulation of the problems to face, in the definition and identification of the possible hazards, in the detection and measurement of the exposure, in the characterization of possible effects. Moreover, explicit normative commitments (i.e. choices shaped by cultural, ethical, economic and political considerations) are made when prioritizing and weighting risks in the cost-benefits analyses (Kastenhofer, 2010).

As Sandra Harding effectively points out (Harding, 2004), the main strategy to defend the standard notion of objectivity, despite this complex and intrinsic blending of facts and values, is to appeal to and make use of a homogeneous epistemic culture: if the values and interests at stake in shaping what is considered as relevant knowledge are shared by the members of the regulatory community, they don't stand out: they are neutral within a seamless background.

Both innovation science and regulatory science are therefore embedded in the modern ideal of "scientists speaking truth to power", and enclosed in an epistemic and normative black box. The closure mechanisms are based on preserving the principles of certainty - in the statistically manageable variant of risk assessment -, objectivity - suitably borrowed from epistemic and normative homogeneity- and exhaustiveness - declined in the form of the lamppost paradox.

3.3 Defending the modern ideal: The three grand narratives of innovation

As we will explore in the following sections, these quite effective stabilizing strategies are supplemented with three "grand narratives" of innovation (Wynne et al., 2008), responsible of reassuring citizens about the "proper" - i.e. modern - functioning of the whole governance system regarding techno-scientific research and implementation. These standardizing narratives can be defined in terms of power, control and urgency. They are in charge of normalizing whatever comes from out of the box, namely complexity, controversy and irreversibility.

The grand narrative of power is rooted in the ideal of scientists as inventors of new entities, committed to extend indefinitely the limits of human being and agency through the creative manipulation of life, energy and matter. Either by reaching new territories on the macro, micro or nano scales, by intervening on organic and inorganic matter, or by converging nano, bio, information and cognitive science technologies, the power of human agency on its surroundings consists on a constant exercise of techno-scientific creative enhancement of the known and prompt treatment of the unknown. In line with the narratives of the green and the blue revolutions, in our context, the narrative of power is directly connected with the issue of food security. Indeed, the "gene revolution" is founded the idea that, with the aid of agri-biotechnology, we can tackle and solve the issue of global hunger, by dramatically increasing our yields and protecting our crops from climatic stresses and diseases. Likewise, with biotechnological aquaculture, we can cheaply provide the needed animal proteins to the hungry world.

Power is nothing without control: safely driving the impressively powerful car of innovation means being able to govern at will the inherent complexity of the interaction between the human techno-scientifically enhanced species and its 'natural' surroundings. In our framework, the narrative of control is declined in terms of (bio)safety, i.e in terms of the capacity to contain the possible health and ecological drawbacks of GMOs, by implementing a variety of barriers (Guarnieri *et al.*, 2008): genetic, ecological, physical, environmental, and last but not least, normative.

Finally, the grand narrative of urgency is based on the assumption of a morally binding necessity to bypass any delaying post-normal knowledge production and decision-making process, in favor of a silver-bullet technoscientific and technocratic approach, in order to effectively confront and solve the pressing socio-environmental problems that afflict the planet, on local and global scales. In this future oriented narrative, lack of time and high stakes produce allegedly compelling mono-causal framings, in which techno-scientific expert knowledge emerge as a "deus ex machina" from the grand narratives of power and control. In other words, in the context of this narrative, one needs to reject any ethical or precautionary controversy about (bio)safety, if one wants to meet the challenge of food security.

In this overall framework, as we will articulate in the following, the main role of precautionary and post-normal science is to confront the epistemic and normative closure of both innovation and regulatory science, attempting to peak in and ultimately to open the black box they are enclosed in.

We will devote the following two sections to explore a variety of relevant open questions raised within the epistemic culture of basic science, in the field of system biology and ecology, starting by analyzing and discussing the fundamental epistemic grounds of the biotechnology enterprise: the central dogma of molecular biology.

4. The central dogma of molecular biology

As we have mentioned, reductionism, determinism and mechanism are the founding pillars of genetic engineering's epistemic culture. According to this view, the ultimate understanding of the living can be attained by reduction to the system's elementary constituents, whose dynamics is simplifiable and from which the whole can be deterministically deduced, that is predicted with certainty. The organisms can then be treated as predictable and controllable mechanisms or, according to the updated version of this metaphor surging from information technologies, as manageable programs. The foundation of corporate biotechnology relies on the normative translation – or, more specifically, of co-production (Jasanoff, 1990 and 2005) - of this paradigm in patenting law: just like any other "novel" and "not-obvious" reproducible mechanical contraption, GMOs are legitimately ascribable to the ontological cosmology of intellectual property rights.

The founding stone of this whole metaphysical (Dupré, 1993), epistemic, and normative structure is the central dogma of molecular biology (Crick, 1958). At the time of its formulation, the dogma appeared to be an extremely solid basis on which the building of new biotechnologies could be constructed. The central dogma is, in itself, relatively simple: the 'genes' are imagined as sequences of nitrogenous bases along the double-stranded DNA helix. The DNA sequences are transcribed into messenger RNA (mRNA) molecules which travel to the sites of protein synthesis where they are translated into a sequence of amino acids (polypeptides or proteins) according to a code – the universal genetic code - which allocates each triplet of nitrogenous bases (codon) a specific amino acid or a stop codon.

By definition, a dogma does not admit exceptions. A scientific dogma describes a regularity in the set of facts by combining two or more categories of observations into what is known as an invariant association. An invariant association allows a significant reduction in the number of particulars needed to describe the perception that we have of reality at that given level. And this is exactly what happened in the formulation of the central dogma, which aims to construct an invariant association – through a hierarchical relationship represented by the one-way flow DNA → RNA → protein – between the nucleic acid category (DNA and RNA) and the protein category. Since, at the time of its formulation, it appeared certain that the relationship between DNA, RNA and protein was always, inevitably the same, the idea of a 'dogma' stuck. The central dogma was, after all, an expression of that golden age of genetics that was the 1950s and the sense of satisfaction that came from having discovered the molecular nature of genes. As Evelyn Fox Keller put it, the dogma, in all its beauty, dazzled minds (Fox Keller, 2001). The double helix soon became the icon of science and DNA the metaphor for the book of life: all that remained to be done was to develop technologies suited to sequencing the genomes of living beings as quickly as possible.

4.1 The Human Genome Project and the crisis of the central dogma

The results recently achieved in the field of genomics have, however, cast doubts over the central dogma, thereby causing a severe crisis in the grounds of genetic engineering's epistemic culture. One of the findings that appeared to be most immediately significant in the conclusions of the human genome project (International Human Genome Sequencing Consortium [IHGSC], 2001; Venter et al., 2001) was the drastic reduction in the estimated number of genes that constitute human genetic make-up: a mere 35,000, that later dropped to 24,000, in any case far fewer than expected (Ast, 2005). The relationship between genome complexity and size was known: a human DNA molecule is 26 times longer than that of a relatively simple organism like yeast (*Saccharomyces cerevisiae*). It was therefore equally likely that the number of codifying human genes was far higher than the 5,800 forming the genetic make-up of yeast. However, gene density, evaluated as the number of codifying genes per million base pairs, was found to be far higher in yeast (483) than in humans (11). This can mean only one thing: the complexity of the organism does not depend on the number of genes, rather on the type and quantity of the DNA sequences that do not code for protein (Ast, 2005). Some 98.5% of the human genome appears to be made of non-coding DNA and only the remaining 1.5% is made up of gene sequences that code for protein (Barbiero, 2004).

The scientific community has now started to realize that the respect for the orthodoxy of the central dogma has caused us to underestimate the non-coding portion of the genome (Shapiro, 2009), known until recently, in that hubris that characterised genetics in the 20th century, as nothing but 'junk' DNA. Here we see how the framing of any specific epistemic culture entails a normative discrimination between relevant knowledge and superfluous epistemic noise.

It is likely than in what we previously considered 'junk', we will find gems of incomparable beauty (Gibbs, 2003a), the key for starting to understand the holarchic nature of genetic information (Barbiero, 2002).

4.2 The hidden molecular layers of genetic information

The central dogma has come to be besieged by a multitude of accompanying problems. It is not the factual evidence that DNA transcribes into RNA or that RNA is translated into protein that is questioned, but the status of dogma and the hierarchical idea implicit to the one-way flow: DNA → RNA → protein. It would undoubtedly be more appropriate to talk about the 'central law of molecular biology' since, by definition, a law of nature describes in more simple terms a highly significant regularity in the set of facts (Ziman, 1984), thereby contemplating a certain number of related exceptions, restrictions and conditions. A special creative commitment is therefore required to update our conceptual tools in order to achieve an overview of molecular genetics that is closer to the empirical evidence brought to light by experimental research. What were originally perceived by scientists as abnormalities and exceptions to the dogma, are increasingly proving to be the manifestations of an extraordinary system of hidden – yet very present and active - layers of genetic information (Ast, 2005; Buiatti Marcello & Buiatti Marco, 2001; Gibbs 2003b; Shapiro, 2009; Storz, 2002; Travis, 2002)[2].

What we referred to as "liminal knowledge" is then fundamental for shifting our view on the living structure and functioning.

4.3 The crisis of genetic engineering's epistemological system

The crisis of the central dogma is entailing the necessity for a deep reconsideration of genetic engineering's epistemic foundations. Contemporary genetic engineering is, indeed, based on the deterministic certainty that the gene product obtained from a sequence of DNA is unique and incontrovertible, i.e. it cannot undergo post-transcriptional modification.

The discovery of hidden molecular layers of genetic information undermines this certainty and makes scientists more aware of the limits of a technology that would need a deep revision. The doubts and questions become pertinent when the uncertainty is such as to condition the outcome of important research programmes. However, in line with what we mentioned so far, this awareness has not been taken on board by regulatory agencies, such as the U.S. Food and Drug Administration (2009).

The genome is proving to be a cosmos apart, dominated by complexity, in which we should move with great caution. Perhaps we are lacking the very conceptual tools needed for exploration: the determinist, reductionist and mechanistic tailor metaphor – the 'cutting and stitching' that is so commonly used amongst biotechnologists – is proving to be excessively simple and misleading (Barbiero, 2002; Dodman et al., 2008). This explains why, after 40 years of promises, embedded in the grand narratives of power and control (Lewontin, 2000),

---

[2] The most significant of these hidden layers include: *Transposons* (McClintock, 1950; Princeton University, 2009; Wicker et al., 2007); *Reverse Transcriptase* (Baltimore, 1970; Skalka & Goff, 1993; Temin & Mizutani, 1970); *RNA interference* (Daneholt, 2006; Ecker & Davis, 1986; Siomi & Siomi , 2009); *RNA editing* (Brennicke et al., 1999; Covello & Gray, 1989; Grosjean & Benne, 1998; Pring et al., 1993); *Mitochondrial Genetic Code* (Elzanowski & Ostell, 2008; Jukes & Osawa, 1990); *Pseudogenes* (Balakirev & Ayala, 2003; Hirotsune et al., 2003; Mighell et al., 2000; Poliseno et al., 2010); *RNA splicing* (Black, 2003; Clancy, 2008; Matlin et al., 2005;); *Riboswitch* (Cheah et al., 2007; Tucker & Breaker, 2005; Vitreschak et al., 2004); and *RNA decoy* (Cesana et al., 2011).

gene therapy sets the pace and continues to be a hope beyond reach. Not that there has been a lack of progress. Quite the opposite, each new piece of knowledge has shed light on an aspect of the system whose complexity we continue to underestimate. Essentially, the more we know the more we realize the vastness of our ignorance about the genome's physiology. We currently have a powerful – albeit anything but refined – instrument for introducing gene sequences into various organisms, however we know next to nothing about what this ability implies within the genome as a whole. And, above all, our experimentation is eminently irreversible: no one knows how to correct possible errors (Camino *et al.*, 2009).

Apparently, all this debate is still placed within the first quadrant of the post-normal diagram, the one of applied science, but, as anticipated, even within the epistemic closure of the laboratory, we are facing the consequences of our direct experimentation on living systems: complexity, irreversibility and controversy dominate our biotechnological endeavour, deeply challenging its epistemic culture. This fact is fraught with consequences both within innovation science, in terms of revising the very idea of the safety and consistency of corporate know-how, and within its regulatory counterpart, in terms of the normative foundations of patenting and on the possibility of quantifying, assessing and managing the impact of our experimentation. All this even before stepping out of the laboratory walls.

Let's now examine some of the main controversial issues related to the impacts of biotechnology in open fields, namely in the agri-food production.

5. GMOs and food production: (Bio)safety, security and the silver-bullet

Research, development and large-scale farming of genetically modified crops are rapidly altering the agriculture scenario worldwide. In 2010, GM seeds worth 11.2 billion US dollars which represents 22% of the global seed market were planted covering a total of 148 million hectares, corresponding to a market value of harvested crops estimated at 150 US dollars (James, 2010).

The proposed benefits of the biotech crop industry vary from specific kinds of resistance - to herbicides, pests and extreme weather conditions - to an enhanced nutritional power, such as the highly controversial Golden Rice, engineered to produce pro-Vitamin A. The possible negative consequences of GM crops for food production include human health issues, negative effects on non-target species and organisms, and irreversible genetic pollution.

In the past few years, GM animals have made their way not only within the pharmaceutical industry – with the emergence of the so-called pharming (Caruso, 2007) –, but also within the food industry. An aquaculture company, the Aqua Bounty Technologies Inc. (ABT), has recently applied for authorization to market a GM Atlantic Salmon as food product for human consumption (Pollack, 2010). In case of approval, this salmon would be the first transgenic animal to be marketed for US dinner tables and it would clear the way for a whole set of redesigns, from fast-growing tilapia and carp (FAO, 2002) to the Enviropig™, engineered to reduce phosphorous pollution (Pollack, 2007; Saenz, 2010).

The making of GMOs for food production introduces a whole new type of ecological hazard, in terms of a possible large-scale and irreversible alteration of genetic information in ecological systems[3]. Indeed, genetically engineered crops have the biological potential to propagate outside of the labile borders of their cultivated fields through seeds, pollens or DNA fragments, with the help of bacteria, and variously interact with other species, both wild and farmed, in their proximity[4]. In the case of aquaculture, as we will later explore, GM fishes could, in principle, evade their breeding infrastructure, and interact with the wild populations, with a very small, but not null, chance of irreversibly altering the eco-systemic balance and the genetic makeup of these latter[5].

As mentioned so far, the structure of the debate around ecological risks of agri-food biotechnology is characterized by the coexistence of different epistemic cultures and strategies, with a variety of normative implications. The innovation science approach is focused on optimizing the products for their declared benefits and on minimizing the deterministically predictable drawbacks. The normative framework of regulatory science is founded on defining dangers in the restricted, quantifiable terms of risks, leaving to precautionary science the burden of proving the existence of possible hazards.

In this scenario, precautionary science is engaged in the arduous task of exploring the complexity of interaction between GMOs and socio-ecological systems, entailing a number of controversial problems.

5.1 Precautionary science open questions

5.1.1 GM crops: Gene flow and introgression

Ecologists are discussing the possibility that a transgene belonging to GM plants could spread to native populations through a process known as introgression – the stable incorporation of a gene in the host genome able to generate a differentiated population. The ecological consequences of a transgene introgression in plants or bacteria are not yet fully understood, but could be significant (Smith & Smith, 2006).

In a recent critical review, we considered vertical and horizontal introgression, we analyzed the biochemical and genetic constraints and the environmental factors that limit the possibility of transgene spread and we illustrated cases in which the natural barriers are overcome (Guarnieri et al., 2008). In the meantime, these concerns have been empirically confirmed, highlighting the relevance of a post-normal framing and management of complexity.

Let's now revisit a crucial debate about introgression, in which precautionary and innovation science had a close and direct confrontation, and a post-normal kind of extended peer review was proven to be essential.

In late 2001, the journal *Nature* published an article by Berkeley scientists Ignatio Chapela and his student David Quist about a possible case of introgression of Bt transgenes in landrace maize, in the Mexican region of Oaxaca, despite the government moratorium on GM maize imposed in 1998 (Quist & Chapela, 2001). The article fuelled a heated debate as it implied that normative barriers were not sufficient to prevent uncontrolled and potentially

---

[3] We will leave aside in this context the possible impacts on human health.
[4] The very notion of 'proximity' is naturally highly controversial in itself (Guarnieri et al., 2008).
[5] For more details, see section 5.1.2 and 5.2.1.

irreversible genetic contamination in the center of origin of this stable crop. In a very short time, *Nature* received a number of outraged criticizing letters, by molecular biologists and biotechnologists, claiming that the results were unacceptable, as the inverse polymerase chain reaction (iPCR) used to amplify and analyze small DNA quantities was extremely sensitive and thus prone to false positives. Chapela's experimental methods were then accused of not meeting the due – i.e. molecular biology - accuracy standards (Kaplinsky *et al.*, 2002; Metz & Fütterer, 2002). One scientist called the paper "a testimony to technical incompetence," another termed it "so outlandish as to be pathetic," and a third dismissed it as "trash and indefensible" (Metz & Parrott, quoted in Lepkowski, 2002). Quist and Chapela's published response was considered inadequate and, although officially only science quality was at stake, the case became rapidly ideologically polarized: the authors were accused of environmentalist biases, their detractors of improperly defending the industrial biotech lobby. The journal itself was forced to justify the whole publication process[6]. As Jasanoff eloquently points out, the article was subject to a greater degree of scrutiny than the crops themselves had undergone in the passage from lab to field to commercial cultivation (Jasanoff, 2005).

As a result, in April 2002, *Nature's* editor Philip Campbell took the unprecedented step of officially withdrawing the journal support to the contested paper, leaving the readers to judge the science for themselves (Campbell, 2002). In this way, for the first time, the subjectivity of scientific judgment under conditions of uncertainty was formally acknowledged in the science community.

Indeed, in this inherently post-normal issue, characterized by lack of full and certain knowledge, the absence of a predefined and agreed upon assessment methodology, the high stakes and the inextricable link between facts and values, the modern-based peer review system was doomed to failure. Although the argument of ideological biases regrettably and improperly occupied the scene, the main issue here is that, when assessing biosafety risks and their potential normative consequences, a level of indeterminacy emerges from the coexistence - and antagonism - between different epistemic cultures, which implicitly legitimate different sampling methods, statistical analyses, and analytical techniques. In this case, the innovation science approach of molecular biology ended up prevailing, with the help of the actual methodological weakness of the Berkeley scientists. A black boxing mechanism was set in place at this point. Indeed, the inadequacy of their sampling methods was incorrectly identified with the actual absence of possible introgression. In other words, the absence of incontrovertible evidence was conveniently identified with the incontrovertible evidence of absence (of introgression), applying the so-called *argomentum ad ignorantiam* (Kastenhofer, 2010).

A later extensive survey performed between 2003 and 2004 in the same region suggested the same line of argument, concluding that transgenic plants were rare or absent in the sampled fields (Ortiz-García *et al.*, 2005). As we have anticipated, the liminal knowledge, typical of precautionary science, can be easily dismissed and normalized.

---

[6] For an extended account of the entire controversy, see Lepkowski (2002), and for an interesting perspective on the ideological charges and delegitimation of the two scientists involved see Monbiot (2002).

It took another four years and the involvement of several different disciplines, such as plant evolutionary ecology, applied statistics, and population ecology to make new measurements, re-examine the 2001 and 2004 samples and find out that the transgenes were indeed present and they had always been there. Interviews with local farmers about seed exchanges indicated that transgenes most likely persisted in the communities after 2001, rather than having been re-introduced. Moreover, new simulation models, based on this experience-based data collection, showed that when pollen and seeds are limited, as in the Oaxaca region, transgenes are likely to be highly aggregated geographically, therefore challenging the statistical methods for calculating the probability of detecting rare events-again liminal knowledge - based on assumptions of random or uniform geographical distributions (Piñeyro-Nelson *et al.*, 2009; Snow, 2009).

Thus, local knowledge was essential for challenging the standard hypotheses of statistical analyses and the experience-based epistemic culture of the scientists involved was crucial for asking the proper questions to the proper agents, namely the local farmers. This decade-long open debate can therefore being interpreted as an illuminating example of how the complexity implied in high power techno-scientific experimentation involves indeterminacy, irreversibility and inherent controversy.

Extended peer community and extended facts, such as the relevant local knowledge of Mexican farmers, was then decisive for re-frame the issue at stake and finding clearer results.

Before exploring the innovation science framing narratives of introgression, let's examine the main biosafety open questions associated with a different type of biotechnological endeavor: the GM salmon.

5.1.2 GM salmon: Trojan gene effect and ethology

ABT succeeded in injecting into the genome of an Atlantic salmon a gene construct constituted by the promoter and termination region from the Ocean Pout (*Zoarces americanus*) antifreeze gene and the growth hormone (GH) gene sequence of Chinook Salmon (*Oncorhynchus tshawytscha*). The corporation has patented the procedure and the resulting fish under the trademark AquAdvantage® Salmon [AAS] (Aqua Bounty Technologies Inc., 2010).

GH stimulates cell division, muscular and skeletal growth, hepatic synthesis of insulin-like growth factor (IGF) and the immune system. GH production is in turn inhibited by the presence of glucocorticoids, which have an anti-inflammatory function, and somatostatin, which inhibits insulin synthesis. In wild-type salmon, the promoter of the gene that regulates GH production is only expressed in response to certain environmental stimuli, such as temperature and the duration of daylight (Bjornsson, 1997), whereas the promoter of genetically modified salmon is continuously active (Devlin *et al.*, 1995). Since gene expression systems are regulated by negative feedback, it would appear clear that the choice of a promoter from a non-*Salmonidae* species has precisely the purpose of preventing the Atlantic Salmon's development regulators from working, thereby effectively isolating the GH production system from the salmon's physiology. The GH of Atlantic Salmon and Chinook salmon are in fact very similar, without being exactly the same. The mRNA nucleotide sequence is 90% identical (1013/1126 nucleotides) and the protein expressed is

94% identical (198/210 amino acids): just 5 amino acids are effectively different (Bodnar, 2010).

During the integration process, the gene construct – known as EO-1α – underwent promoter rearrangement, which reduced its expression potential. Despite this, when the transgenic salmon was backcrossed to a wild-type Atlantic Salmon, the EO-1α gene construct appeared to be stable in the second (F2) and fourth (F4) generations (Yaskowiak et al., 2006). The data released by ABT – which, despite being devoid of independent review (Veterinary Medicine Advisory Committee - Food and Drug Administration Center for Veterinary Medicine [VMAC], 2010), was accepted as reliable by scientific literature (Fox, 2010) – show that AAS gains weight about 3 times faster than wild-type Atlantic Salmon (Aqua Bounty Technology Inc., 2010). The idea is then to develop a fish product that is materially equivalent to its wild-type counterpart, but it is functionally different, namely more efficient, as it requires less time to grow and be ready for the market.

The evaluation of the risks and impacts of this techno-scientific experimentation is highly controversial and some of the main issues raised within the precautionary science framework involve again possible ecological hazards, emerging from the relations between the communities of GM and wild-type salmon. The debate hinges around two questions: whether the transgene's presence alters the fitness of the GM salmon compared to that of the wild-type salmon and what happens if a GM salmon mixes with a wild-type population. Three main topics of experimental investigation can therefore be defined: (1) the possible competition between GM and wild-type populations; (2) the potential transfer of the transgene to the wild-type population; and (3) the evaluation of the predatory behavior of the GM salmon on the wild-type homologue.

Since the assessment of fitness in natural environments is difficult to assess experimentally, a number of theoretical models have been developed. One of the most interesting is the one devised by Muir & Howard (1999), who articulated the "Trojan Gene Effect", where the mingling of the populations of GM salmon with the wild-type salmon populations can lead to increases or decreases in GM salmon fitness, however, in both cases to the detriment of the ecosystem. In another theoretical model, the increase in frequency of the GM genotypes in any case corresponds to a reduction in the fitness of the wild-type population (Hendrick, 2001). When considered together, these models, show that the GM salmon can also have poorer overall fitness than its wild-type homologue, that is often related to malformations and physiological problems of various kinds (Deitsch et al., 2006; Eales et al., 2004; Hu & Zhu, 2010; Leggat et al., 2007; Roberts et al., 2004). In any case, when a GM salmon is introduced into a natural environment, the modelled risk is that it will lead to the extinction of the wild type.

These theoretical models are backed by a number of experimental papers. Various studies indicate that the GM salmon are effectively less fit, either because they grow too fast (Devlin et al., 1994; Devlin et al., 1995) or because mortality rises in certain conditions, such as the presence of predators or a shortage of food (Sundström et al., 2004). However, in natural conditions, what are the real availabilities of food for any escaped GM Salmon? Sundström et al. (2007) compared salmon raised in tanks with salmon raised in an environment simulating natural conditions. The GM Coho Salmon grow larger, up to three times longer than the wild type. In pseudo-natural conditions they only grow 20% longer. In this context, it is interesting to consider the findings of Devlin *et al.* (2004), who report that when the GM salmon are raised in the same tanks as the wild type, they live together peacefully whilst there is plenty of food. However, when food becomes scarce, the GM salmons demonstrate dominant behavior, and even cannibalism, thereby leading to the extinction of both populations. In the same food shortage conditions, the wild-type salmon would have survived without any real problem.

In general, all these studies point out a recurrent issue in the precautionary science epistemic approach: even minimal changes to the initial conditions can lead to very different results that are difficult to compare, thereby making it arduous to evaluate the risk associated with the introduction of the GM salmon into aquatic ecosystems in experimental conditions.

5.2 Innovation science normalizing strategies

5.2.1 The narrative of control: (Bio)safety and the myth of containment

In light of what we have experienced so far, the phenomena of gene flow and introgression are highly complex and controversial. Nonetheless, a powerful narrative of control, based on the notion of barrier is dominating the innovation and regulatory framework.

A clear example in which the lack of knowledge involved in open field biotech experimentation was reduced to statistically manageable risk assessment, is a study by the American plant biologist and biotechnologist Neal Stewart, later extended in a book for the general public (Stewart, 2003; 2004). The vertical (i.e sexual) introgression phenomenon is subdivided in a finite and numerable set of discreet steps that can be isolated and individually analyzed. These steps are essentially the minimum known linear cause-effect conditions under which gene introgression can occur between any given GM plant and a relative population. In order to overcome these natural barriers the two species must: (1) be sexually compatible, (2) grow near one another, and (3) have partially overlapping flowering times. Moreover, (4) the first generation F1 hybrids must persist for at least one generation and be sufficiently fertile to produce backcross hybrids (BC1). Finally (5) the transgene must have a selective advantage for the wild relative and (6) backcross generations must progress to the point at which the transgene is incorporated into the genome of the wild relative. Each barrier depends on a limited number of variables and interactions. Moreover, a one-to-one correspondence can be established between any given barrier and a corresponding probability distribution of being crossed (Guarnieri *et al.*, 2008). This determinist, reductionist and mechanist approach extend the epistemic culture of innovation science from the controlled *in vitro* regime, to the complex *in vivo* open field. The crucial normative implication of this framing is the possibility of applying specific counter-measures, allowing for regulatory principles – such as the European framework of co-existence (Commission of the European Communities, 2003) - and consequent modeling and policy implementations based on environmental and geographical confinement (Commission of the European Communities, 2006). Moreover, this biotech framing allows for the implementation of genetic barriers in the secured laboratory set up, in terms of programmed seed sterilization, through the highly controversial Gene Use Restriction Technology (GURT) methods. These sterilizing methods, born as normative barriers for copyright protection and highly contested by the civil society as forms of commons misappropriation (Shiva, 1997)[7], are therefore recycled as techno-scientific barriers, in the scenario of risk management.

Let's now move to the GM salmon case, in which the same kind of framing is applied.

In a recent report on the risk assessment and mitigation of AquAdvantage Salmon (Bodnar, 2010), the complex and controversial biosafety issue of possible genetic flow and perturbation in wild populations, is reduced to the implementation of a series of counter-measures, namely biological, physical and environmental barriers, characterized by a statistically quantifiable margin of uncertainty, as emerging from the laboratory set up and procedures.

The first biological barrier consists in breeding only sterile all-female salmons. Sterility is achieved by triploid induction through pressure shock (Benfey, 1988). Indeed, having three copies of each chromosome, triploids fishes cannot produce gametes and therefore they are sterile. Nonetheless, the percentage of infertility induction is never certain (Devlin, 2010) and moreover triploid fishes grow slower (Devlin, 2004) and have a higher chance of manifesting aberrant phenotypes (VMAC, 2010). In ABT laboratories, the success rate of this techniques is guaranteed at 98,9%, leaving only 1,1% diploid eggs. Nonetheless, some concerns emerge in the ABT report, as they feel the need to explicitly declare that each sterilized eggs batch will be sampled and destroyed if the diploid eggs percentage is 5% or more (Aqua Bounty Technology, 2010). AquAdvantage salmon genetic females that are homozygous for the EO-1α gene are induced with 17-methyltestosterone to produce male gonads (neomales). The male gametes (deriving from chromosomic females and therefore without male chromosomes) so produced are used to fertilize wild type salmon eggs. As a result, all newborns are females, with a copy of the EO-1α gene (Bodnar, 2010).

Given the small, but existing probability (1.1% at most) of diploids salmons being grown, ABT plans to isolate the structure through a number of physical barriers, such as fencing, on-facility living quarters for security personnel, 24 hours a day surveillance with the help of security cameras, plus filters, nets and other containment device. Here, biosafety becomes a matter of surveillance, directly borrowing the real and metaphoric epistemic culture of security services, contrasting techno-scientific uncertainty with active control measures. But, like any other of this kind, such a complex and expensive system is inherently prone to accidents, as indeed documented in a vast literature about Atlantic Salmon's escapes (Crozier, 1998; Gausen & Moen, 1991; McKinnell *et al.*, 1997).

Finally, the AquAdvantage Salmon land-based production facilities are located in Canada (Prince Edward Island) and in Panama, where a number of environmental barriers are already in place. The fresh bodies of water of eastern Canada have been one of the natural habitats of Atlantic Salmon. But today this fish is extinct, due to overexploitation, acid rain and barriers to migration. According the ABT, in case of escape, AquAdvantage Salmon would find the same environmental problems that drove its wild counterpart to extinction (Bodnar, 2010). Nonetheless, even if highly degraded, those waters are indeed salmon's natural habitat. On the other hand, in Panama, the facility is located at a high altitude, near a river that drains to the Pacific Ocean. Much of the river water is utilized for power

---

[7] The most famous patent associated with this kind of transgenic technique was quite ineffectively called Terminator and rapidly withdrawn from the market (US Patent 5, 723, 765, 1998).

generation and the numerous canals that control water flow to power generation facilities are not suitable for salmons. Moreover the river water is used up to a 100% for 4-5 months a year. The nearby waters could sustain a young salmon for some time but the elevated water temperatures near the ocean would make it very hard to survive. Escape to the Pacific Ocean is therefore highly unlikely (Bodnar, 2010).

As we can see, a principle of deterministically controlled redundancy is used to ideally, asymptotically, reduce the unavoidable presence of uncertainty. However, as was demonstrated in the case of GM crops introgression, even if barriers are strict and redundant, in accordance with the law of large numbers, over long term and for large populations, they are inevitably overcome (Guarnieri *et al.*, 2008). Moreover, in this overall "lamppost" paradoxical scenario, indeterminacy and ignorance are completely dismissed, as not "scientifically" - i.e. statistically - manageable, and thus not functional to the modern framing of regulatory processes.

5.2.2 The narrative of power: Food security and the myth of enhanced yield

The issue of (bio)safety has been threatening the successful introduction of GM crops in the food production system since the beginning, in the early-nineties. Moreover, in the then globalizing market, the biotech industry had to face the difficult task of confronting its products with a variety of cultural, political, historical and economic configurations, belonging to the different targeted affluent countries. Overall, these patterns were converging in diversified civic epistemologies, implying contrasting epistemic and normative framings of the biotechnological endeavor (Jasanoff, 2005).

While the established regulatory notion of substantial equivalence[8] (OECD, 1993) was ensuring a fast expansion in the US market, when the move was made across the Atlantic Ocean, GM products encountered a strong opposition in European countries, related to a number of factors, including the threat of losing market shares and the relatively fresh memory of the BSE food safety shock (Ibrahim, 1996). In 1998, The European Union resolved to adopt a precautionary approach and impose a moratorium on new biotechnological products. This decision challenged the US export patterns and opened new kinds of regulatory oversight within the globalized free market set up of the WTO.

Around the same time, in a quite unsettling circular loop, the biotech industry was facing raising concerns back in the US. In 1999, a new heated biosafety controversy regarding possible adverse effects on non-target insects (Losey, 1999) appeared in the news media. Indeed, disturbingly evoking Rachel Carson "silent spring" (Carson, 1962), the potentially 'innocent victims' of GM Bt cotton were the highly symbolically beautiful monarch butterflies, whose images and costumes ended up dominating the scene at the 1999 anti-globalization riots that occurred in Seattle and Washington, USA.

---

[8] Endorsed by the FAO and the WHO in the early 1990s, the notion of substantial equivalence essentially frames the food safety regulatory process in the controversial reductionist terms of biochemical profiling. This type of assessment reduces the costs- and the time-to market of GM food products. Born as a compromise between science and the market the substantial equivalence principle was assumed by the law as a certain scientific procedure, grounding in this way the consequential normative justification for not labeling GM foods as such in the USA (Tallacchini, 2000).

Strong counter-measures were thus needed (Barboza, 1999) and a renewed effort was made by the main biotechnology corporations to emphasize the potential benefits of their genetically engineered food products. A number of industry-wide alliances were set in place at that time - such as the Alliance for Better Foods - financing scientific research, organizing educational forums, lobbying legislators, regulators and farms organizations and using their own web sites to promote the benefits of GM products (www.betterfoods.org). In this way, a narrative of power took shape and was diffused through specialized literature, as well as the mass media (Fernandez-Cornejo & Caswell, 2006; McLaren, 2005). Great expectations were placed on the capacity of the emerging biotech industrial production system to improve crop yields and, in the very near future, to provide nutritionally enhanced food products, such as the Golden Rice, which made the cover picture of Time Magazine in 2000, and initiated a still ongoing scientific, regulatory and cultural controversy (Time, 2000; Pollan, 2001; Potrykus, 2010).

In response to biosafety concerns, this narrative of power brushed up the questionable Malthusian assumption that correlates hunger with a gap between food production and population growth, shifting in this way the attention to the issue of global food security. In line with a culturally granted endorsement of the "green revolution", considered in that context as a key innovation triumph in the agri-food system, the prospects of genetic engineering applied to food production were purposefully named as "gene revolution". Not only this upgraded techno-scientific application would raise agricultural productivity, but also it would significantly help to reduce the chemical inputs, cleaning up some of the main inconveniences of the previous version.

Twenty years later, an extensive review by the Union of Concerned Scientists on the actual aggregate yield improvement in the US agriculture system reveals quite a different scenario about the alleged promises genetic engineering (Union of Concerned Scientists, 2009).

The report evaluates in detail the intrinsic and the operational yield of two primary GE food and feed crops, namely corn and soy. Intrinsic yield, the highest that can be achieved, is obtained when crops are grown under ideal conditions; it may also be thought of as potential yield. By contrast, operational yield is obtained under field conditions, when environmental factors such as pests and stress result in yields that are considerably less than ideal. Genes that improve operational yield reduce losses from such factors. In order to live up to the food security challenge, not only potential but also intrinsic yield has to be improved. The key finding of the analysis is that the raising of intrinsic yields, both of soy and corn, during the twentieth century are not ascribable to the genetically engineered traits but to the successes of traditional breeding. Concurrently, out of several thousand field trials, many of which have been intended to raise operational and intrinsic yield, only Bt corn has succeeded and only as far as operational yield. Moreover, the gains delivered were minimal compared to the overall gains within non GM crops: insect-resistant Bt corn varieties have provided an average yield advantage of 3-4% compared to conventional practices, but overall the conventional breeding methods have increased yields of the major crops of 13-25% (Union of Concerned Scientists, 2009).

As to the prospects for the future, the report interestingly argues that, even granting the very optimistic possible margin of a 50% yield increase, estimated by theoretical research on the limitations of plant physiology and morphology, the actual projections for the potential contribution of genetic engineering should take into account the fact that most of the transgenes under current exam may succeed in raising intrinsic yield, but may never reach the market. Indeed, these second-generation GMOs are characterized by greater intrinsic genetic complexity: unlike the ones currently commercialized, they have the potential to influence a number of other genes, therefore entailing multiple and unpredictable side effects on a crop. The systemic approach of precautionary science and the crisis of the central dogma suggest that, once again, ignorance and indeterminacy are highly significant and would require, as the report recommends, a radical revision of the regulatory processes involved. Thus, keep betting on genetic engineering for addressing food security will have unavoidable consequences in terms of food (bio)safety. Clearly, the objection coming from the epistemic culture of innovation is that these new possible harmful side effects will be managed through more powerful risk assessment technologies and will be effectively balanced with the needed countermeasures. Once more, we see how the black boxing mechanism can be at work and how these two narratives of innovation, control and power, are closely depending on one another.

A fully analogous line of argument can be retraced in the case of GM salmons. In this context, the narrative of power rests on further enhancing the alleged remarkable performances of the aquaculture "blue revolution" (Vassallo et al., 2007) and on tackling the issue of food security by effectively responding to the globally growing need for healthy and cheap animal proteins. Again, indefinite (bio)safety risks are explicitly weighted up against definite food security benefits. In a recent article published on the journal Science (Smith et al., 2010), a whole dissertation on US salmon market aggregate prices is made, arguing that the FDA regulatory processes should take charge of the changing patterns of animal protein consumption, induced by technologically driven declining costs. In particular, for a "full impact assessment" of GM salmons, the regulatory agency should compare the possible minor nutritional and health drawbacks of GM fishes, with the major substantial public health benefits of eating more salmon instead of other proteins, such as beef. In this context, the AquAdvantage salmon is reductionistically framed as a product: in terms of its alleged lower production and market costs – a benefit of being GM - and of its healthier nutritional power – a benefit of being substantially equivalent to a wild type salmon. Both statements are endorsed as evidence-based, i.e. objective, within the black boxing innovation and regulatory epistemic culture. The framing data statements such as: "For American adults eating no fish, consumption of just one serving of salmon per week can reduce coronary death of 36%", are as narrowly selected as purposefully effective (Smith et al., 2010).

5.2.3 The narrative of urgency: The silver-bullet for global hunger

Having set in place a narrative of control - in charge of defending (bio)safety - and a narrative of power - in charge of enhancing food security-, a third fundamental narrative of innovation was developed, in order to make GM products, not only safe and desirable but also urgently needed.

At the turn of the century, world leaders pledged to halve hunger and extreme poverty by 2015, as the first of eight fundamental Millennium Development Goals (MDG). The UN Millennium Declaration, adopted by 189 nations, provided a specific timeframe for measuring results and draw public attention to the issue of global food security. In the meantime, in the affluent world, the biotechnological food market was relatively confined to North America, given the Mexican moratorium on corn and the European ban on new GM products, as we have seen, both established in 1998. The so-called developing countries represented a large and less regulated market-share to occupy. A new form of controversy was then emerging, again between different epistemic and normative cultures, about the role of genetic engineering in tackling and solving the problem of global hunger. The founding assumptions of the innovation approach can be located in an extensive report by the Consultative Group on International Agricultural Research, published in 1999 (CGIAR, 1999): given the major socio-economic differences between the countries where the debate about GMOs is taking place and the countries where they are actually needed, the positions and the conclusions of the formers are largely irrelevant to the latter (Persley, in CGIAR, 1999). Moreover, a silver-bullet high-power technology is needed to fight the enemies of health and wealth. In Gabrielle Persley's words: "The innovation science of molecular biology and other tools of biotechnology add elegance and precision to the pursuit of solutions to thwart poverty, malnutrition, and food insecurity in too many countries around the world. In agriculture, these enemies are manifest as pests, diseases, drought and other biotic and abiotic stresses that limit the productivity of plants and animals" (Persley, in CGIAR, 1999, p. 3).

Risks and benefits of genetically engineered food processes and products should be thus weighted against the urgent needs of the poor. The regulatory debate was to be considered as a privilege of affluent nations, not applicable to developing world: where extreme poverty and hunger are prevalent discussing about uncertainty is a luxury that can't be afforded.

A study published in 2004, on the environmental (bio)safety of a transgenic nematode resistant variety of potato, documented gene flow towards wild relatives that grow in the proximity (Celis et al., 2004). The problem was deepened by the fact that the transgenic variety was grown in one of the most important areas of biodiversity conservation (The Central Andes), where 130 wild species of potatoes that are sexually compatible with transgenic crops had been documented. The similarity with the Chapela case could have initiated a similar long-term controversy. Nonetheless, the scientists who conducted this research followed the Nuffield Council of Bioethics position, whereby the risk of compromising biodiversity by introgression is not a sufficient reason for banning the use of GM crops in developing countries, where a response to denutrition (Nuffield Council on Bioethics, 2004) is an urgent issue. "The Nuffield Council on Bioethics, suggests that introgression of genetic material into related species in centres of crop biodiversity is an insufficient justification to ban the use of genetically modified crops in the developing world. They consider that a precautionary approach to forgo the possible benefits invokes the fallacy of thinking that doing nothing is itself without risk to the poor" (Celis et al., 2004, p. 223). As we can see, the main argument is founded on a dualistic normative approach according to which either we deploy the most advanced techno-scientific implementation, i.e. the silver-bullet, regardless of the possible (bio)safety consequences, or they are left with nothing.

This technocratic normative assumption can be found in the Nuffield Council on Bioethics' actual recommendation: "[...] it is easier to forgo possible benefits in the light of assumed hazards, if the existing *status quo* is already largely satisfactory. Thus, for developed countries, the benefits offered by GM crops may, so far, be relatively modest. However, in developing countries the degree of poverty and the often unsatisfactory state of health and agricultural sustainability is the baseline and the feasibility of alternative ways to improve their situation must be the comparator" (Nuffield Council on Bioethics, 2004, p. 58). In 2004, a few years have passed already from the first optimistic statements about future yield increase and in affluent countries the food security arguments are not as effective. In the Nuffield Council's vision, yield enhancement may not be so significant in our context, but in the developing countries, it still have to prioritized over (bio)safety. As a result, the narrative of urgency can then be interpreted as an effective epistemic and normative strategy to fill up the gaps of both the narrative of control and of power[9].

6. Concluding remarks: From predicting risks to diagnosing needs

As we have seen, when applying genetic engineering to our food production system, we are faced with emergent and irreducible complexity, implying the presence of ignorance and indeterminacy. Moreover, as articulated earlier (see section 2), our direct and high-power experimentation can be considered as fundamentally irreversible with unknown long term consequences.

The impact of these biotechnologies has been, and still is, prominently evaluated in terms of possible future consequences and the latter are in turn declined in the restrictive framework of quantifiable risks and benefits. So far, we have explored the fundamental epistemic and normative limits of risks assessments in this context, and the normalizing strategies to keep them operational.

We would like to conclude our reflections by concentrating on the logically former, fundamental premise of this whole framework of analysis, namely the strong and implicit normative stance according to which we identify impact evaluation with future developments. This assumption is the grounding pillar of the modern principle of responsibility, according to which we need to predict the future in order to justify our action in the present (Funtowicz & Strand, 2011).

When fully acknowledged, the complexity and irreversibility of our techno-scientific experimentation lead necessarily to a revision of this principle. Indeed, we are left in the paradoxical situation in which we need to know about the future consequences of our implementation in order to act, but we are prevented from knowing the future developments, as a consequence of the intrinsic nature of the very same implementation (Benessia et al., 2012). A way out of this inherent contradiction is to shift our attention back to the present and to divert our analytical and reflective capacity from prediction to diagnose and from responsibility under risk to commitment in times of change (Funtowicz & Strand, 2011).

Sheila Jasanoff articulates this kind of paradigm change by advocating the need for new "technologies of humility", directed to alleviate known causes of people's vulnerability to harm, to openly address the issue of equity and the socio-economical realignments implied by the new emergent technologies, and to reflect on the social factors that promote or discourage learning from our (technological) past and present experience (Jasanoff, 2003; 2008).

---

[9] A more recent version of this narrative of urgency is applied to the climate change emergency, in terms of both mitigation and adaptation.

When applied to our case study, this approach actually allows opening up the black box of the overall narratives of innovation, and reconsidering the whole biotechnology enterprise as the tip of the iceberg of the industrial agriculture and breeding main paradigm – the basis of the green and the blue revolution - with all its long-term inherently dysfunctional properties.

Indeed, this model of food production is based on the linearization of flows of nutrients, requiring a progressive depletion of stocks – such as fossil energy, soil erosion, loss of biodiversity – and the progressive filling of sinks – in terms of environmental pollution and greenhouse gasses (Folke et al., 1998; Giampietro, 2009). Moreover, the prime purpose of this paradigm is to maximize production and to increase efficiency – accordingly defined in the restrictive terms of quantity and total output -, temporarily externalizing social, cultural and environmental costs. In fact, augmenting efficiency in this context intrinsically collide with the preservation of diversity, and therefore of flexibility and adaptability, the two main evolutionary strategies for a sound long-term stability of terrestrial ecosystems (Giampietro, 1994).

In more concrete terms, in order to maximize efficiency, industrial agriculture and breeding increasingly replaces traditional biological varieties with hybrid seeds and breeds - produced by a few big commercial corporations - and traditional knowledge and practices with standardized, corporate techno-scientific know-how.

This transformation necessarily reduces our collective natural resilience and progressively forces our reliance on further (bio)technological fixes, alimenting yet another – destructive - Catch 22 situation. The modern narratives of control, power and urgency applied to the agri-food biotechnology enterprise are embedded in this sterile epistemic and normative circular loop, and therefore they lead to unsustainable processes.

Once again, a way out of the paradox is to reconsider our relation with food and food production altogether and move to a more complex model (Waltner-Toews & Lang, 2000), in which what we eat is not defined in the generic terms of yet another commodity, nor in the reductionist terms of needed calories and nutrients, but it is embedded in a democratized constellation of social, cultural and ecological public values. In other words, we need to move from food (bio)safety and security assessment to a complex and democratic food quality evaluation.

7. References

Altieri, M.A., & Rosset, P. (1999) Ten reasons why biotechnology will not ensure food security, protect the environment and reduce poverty in the developing world, AgBioForum, Vol. 2, n. 3-4, pp. 155-162.

Aqua Bounty Technologies, Inc. (2010) Environmental assessment for AquAdvantage salmon. 26.08.2011, Available from:
http://www.fda.gov/downloads/AdvisoryCommittees/CommitteesMeetingMaterials/VeterinaryMedicineAdvisoryCommittee/UCM224760.pdf

Ast, G. (2005) The Alternative Genome, Scientific American, Vol. 292, pp. 40-47 (April 2005).

Balakirev, E.S., & Ayala, F.J. (2003) Pseudogenes: are they "junk" or functional DNA? Annu. Rev. Genet., Vol. 37, pp. 123–51.

Baltimore, D. (1970) Viral RNA-dependent DNA Polymerase: RNA-dependent DNA Polymerase in Virions of RNA Tumour Viruses. *Nature* Vol. 226, pp. 1209-1211.

Barbiero, G. (2002) Il DNA leggero. *Naturalmente*, Vol. 15, n. 2, pp. 14-19.

Barbiero, G. (2004) *Il principio di precauzione nella crisi dell'impianto epistemologico dell'ingegneria genetica*. Università del Sacro Cuore, Centro di Ricerche per lo Sviluppo Sostenibile della Lombardia. 21.03.2012. Available from: http://www.crasl.unicatt.it/pubblicazioni/CRASL-025-S12-2004.pdf

Barbiero, G., Colucci Gray, L., Camino, E., Guarnieri, V., & Benessia, A. (2011) A real full impact assessment of the genetically modified salmon. *Proceedings of the XXI Congress of the Italian Society of Ecology* (SItE), Palermo, October 3-6, 2011, p. 64.

Barboza, D. (1999) Biotech companies take on critics of gene-altered food. *The New York Times*, November 12, 1999.

Beck, U. (1992) *Risk society: towards a new modernity*. London: Sage

Benessia, A. (2009) From certainty to complexity: science and technology in a democratic society. In Gray, D., Colucci-Gray, L., & Camino, E. (Eds.) *Science Society and Sustainability: Education and Empowerment for an Uncertain World*, New York: Routledge.

Benessia, A., Funtowicz, S. *et al.* (2012). Hybridizing sustainability: Towards a new praxis for the present human predicament. *Sustainability Science*, Vol.7, No.1, pp.75-89.

Benfey, T.J., Bosa, P.G., Richardson, N.L., & Donaldson, E.M.. (1988) Effectiveness of a commercial-scale pressure shocking device for producing triploid salmonids. *Aquacul. Engineer.* Vol. 7, pp. 147-154.

Björnsson, B.T. (1997) The biology of salmon growth hormone: from daylight to dominance. *Fish Physiology and Biochemistry Vol.* 17, pp. 9-24.

Black, D. L. (2003) Mechanisms of alternative pre-messenger RNA splicing. *Annual Reviews of Biochemistry*, Vol.72, No.1, pp. 291-336.

Bodansky, D. (1994) The precautionary principle in US environmental law. In: O'Riordan, T., Cameron, J. (eds.), *Interpreting the Precautionary Principle*, London: Earthscan, pp. 203- 228.

Bodnar, A. (2010) Risk Assessment and Mitigation of AquAdvantage Salmon. *Information Systems for Biotechnology News Report*, pp. 1-7.

Brennicke, A., Marchfelder, A., & Binder, S. (1999) RNA editing. *FEMS Microbioliogy Reviews*, Vol. 23, n. 3, pp. 297-316.

Buiatti, Marcello, & Buiatti, Marco (2001) The Living State of Matter. *Rivista di Biologia / Biology Forum*, Vol. 94, pp. 59-82.

Butler, D., & Reichhardt, T. (1999) Long-term effect of GM crops serves up food for thought. *Nature*, Vol. 398, pp. 651-653.

Camino, E., Barbiero, G., Perazzone, A., & Colucci Gray, L. (2005) Linking research and education to promote an integrated approach to sustainability, Chapter 21 of the *Handbook of Environmental Education, Communication and Sustainability*, Walter Leal Filho (ed.), Frankfurt am Main: Peter Lang GmbH, ISBN 3-631-52606-7, pp. 535-562.

Camino, E., Barbiero, G., & Marchetti, D. (2009) Science Education for Sustainability. Teaching Learning Processes with Science Researchers and Trainee Teachers. In D. Gray, L. Colucci Gray and E. Camino (eds). *Science, Society and Sustainability: Education and Empowerment for an Uncertain World* (Chapter 6). Milton Park, UK: Routledge, pp. 119-153.

Campbell, P. (2002) Editorial note. *Nature*, Vol. 416, p. 601.

Carson R. (1962). *Silent Spring*, Boston: Houghton Mifflin.

Caruso, D. (2007) How to confine the plants of the future? *The New York Times*. April 8.

Cesana, M., Cacchiarelli, D., Legnini, I., Santini, T., Sthandler, O., Chinappi, M., Tramontano, A., & Bozzoni, I. (2011) A long noncoding RNA controls muscle differentiation by functioning as a competing endogenous RNA. *Cell* Vol. 147, pp. 358-369.

Celis, C., M. Scurrah, S. Cowgill, S. Chumbiauca, J. Green, J. Franco, et al. (2004) Environmental biosafety and transgenic potato in a centre of diversity for this crop. *Nature*, Vol. 432, pp. 222-225.

Cheah, M.T., Wachter, A.,, Sudarsan, N., & Breaker, R.R. (2007) Control of alternative RNA splicing and gene expression by eukaryotic riboswitches. *Nature*, Vol. 447, pp. 497–500.

Clancy, S. (2008) RNA Splicing: Introns, Exons and Spliceosome. *Nature Education* 1 (1). 14.10.2011. Available from: www.nature.com/scitable/topicpage/rna-splicing-introns-exons-and-spliceosome-12375

Colucci Gray, L., Camino, E., Barbiero, G., & Gray, D. (2006), From scientific literacy to sustainability literacy: An Ecological Framework for Education. *Science Education*, Vol. 90, pp. 227-252.

Colucci Gray, L., Benessia, A., Guarnieri, V., Barbiero, G., & Camino, E. (2011) From tissues with nanoparticles to transgenic salmons. Which competences for educating civil society to sustainability? *Culture della Sostenibilità*, Vol. 8, pp. 190-205.

Commission of the European Communities (2000) *Communication from the Commission on the Precautionary Principle*. Brussel 2.2.2000, COM(2000)

Commission of the European Communities (2003) *Commission Recommendation on guidelines for the development of national strategies and best practices to ensure the coexistence of genetically modified crops with conventional and organic farming*. Brussel 23.7.2003 (2003/556/EC).

Commission of the European Communities, JRC, European Science and Technology Observatory (2006) *New case studies on the coexistence of GM and non-GM crops in European agriculture*. EUR 22102 EN.

Consultative Group on International Agricultural Research (CGIAR) (1999), *Agricultural Biotechnology and the Poor: Conference Papers*, October. 12/11/2011. Available from: www.cgiar.org/publications/agribiotech.html

Covello, P.S., & Gray, M.W. (1989) RNA editing in plant mitochondria. *Nature*, Vol.341, No.6243, pp. 662–666.

Crick, F. (1958) Central Dogma of Molecular Biology. *Nature*, Vol.227, pp. 661-663.

Crozier, W.W. (1998) Incidence of escaped farmed salmon, *Salmo salar L.*, in commercial salmon catches and fresh water in Northern Ireland. *Fish. Manage. Ecol.*, Vol. 5, pp. 23–29.

Daneholt, B. (2006) Advanced Information: RNA interference. *The Nobel Prize in Physiology or Medicine 2006*. 12.10.2011. Available from: http://nobelprize.org/nobel_prizes/medicine/laureates/2006/adv.html.

Deitch, E.J. Fletcher, G.L., Petersen, L.H., Costa, I.A.S.F., Shears, M.A., Driedzic, W.R., & Gamperl, A.K. (2006) Cardiorespiratory modifications, and limitations, in postsmolt growth hormone transgenic Atlantic salmon *Salmo salar*. *Journal of Experimental Biology*, Vol. 209, pp. 1310-1325.

De Marchi, B. & Ravetz, J. (1999) Risk management and governance: a post-normal science approach. *Futures*, Vol.31, No.7, pp.743-757.

Devlin, R.H., Yesaki, T.Y., Biagi, C.A., Donaldson, E.M., Swanson, P., & Chen, W.K. (1994) Extraordinary salmon growth. *Nature*, Vol. 371, n. 1994, pp. 209-210.

Devlin, R.H., Yesaki, T.Y., Donaldson, E.M., Bu, S.J., & Hew C.L. (1995) Production of germline transgenic Pacific salmonids with dramatically increased growth performance. *Canadian J of Fisheries and Aquatic Sci, Vol.* 52, n. 7, pp. 1376-1384.

Devlin, R.H., Biagi, C.A., & Yesaki, T.Y. (2004) Growth, viability and genetic characteristics of GH transgenic coho salmon strains. *Aquaculture*, Vol. 236, pp. 607-632.

Devlin, R.H. (2010) Occurrence of incomplete paternal-chromosome retention in GH-transgenic coho salmon being assessed for reproductive containment by pressure-shock-induced triploidy. *Aquacolture* Vol. 304, pp. 66-78.

Dodman, M., Camino, E. & Barbiero, G. (2008) Language and Science: products and processes of signification in the educational dialogue. *Journal of Science Communication, Vol* 7, n.3, A01. 28.08.2011. Available from: http://jcom.sissa.it/archive/07/03/Jcom0703%282008%29A01/

Eales, J.G., Devlin, R., Higgs, D.A., McLeese, J.M., Oakes, J.D., & Plohman, J. (2004) Thyroid function in growth-hormone-transgenic coho salmon (*Oncorhynchus kisutch*). *Canadian Journal of Zoology* Vol. 82, n. 8, pp. 1225-1229.

Ecker, J.R., & Davis, R.W. (1986) Inhibition of gene expression in plant cells by expression of antisense RNA. *Proc Natl Acad Sci USA*, Vol. 83, n. 15, pp. 5372–5376.

Elser, J., & Bennet, E. (2011) A broken biogeochemical cycle, *Nature*, Vol. 478, pp. 29-31.

Elzanowski, A., & Ostell, J. (2008) The Genetic Codes. National Center for Biotechnology Information. 29.10.2011. Available from: http://www.ncbi.nlm.nih.gov/Taxonomy/Utils/wprintgc.cgi?mode=c.

European Environmental Agency (2001) *Late lessons from early warnings: the precautionary principle 1986-2000*. Available from http://www.eea.eu.int

FAO (2002) *Biotechnology in food and agriculture*, Conference 7, Available from: http://www.fao.org/biotech/C7doc.htm

Fernandez-Cornejo, J., & Caswell, M. (2006) The first decade of genetically engineered crops in the United States. *Economic Research Service, Economic Information Bulletin*, n. 11. Washington, DC: U.S. Department of Agriculture.

Folke C., Kautsky N., Berg H, Jansson Å, & Troell M. (1998) The ecological footprint concept for sustainable seafood production: a review. *Ecological Applications*, Vol.8, n.1, supplement, pp. S63–S71, by the Ecological Society of America

Fox, J.L. (2010) Transgenic salmon inches toward finish line. *Nature Biotechnology*, Vol. 28, n. 11, pp. 1141-1142.

Fox Keller, E. (2000) *The Century of the Gene*, Harvard MS: Harvard University Press.

Francescon, S. (2006) The impact of GMOs on poor countries: a threat to the achievement of the millennium development goals? *Rivista di Biologia / Biology Forum*, Vol. 99, pp. 381-394.

Funtowicz, S., & Ravetz, J. (1990) *Uncertainty and quality in science for policy*. Dordrecht NL: Kluver Academics Publishers.

Funtowicz, S., & Ravetz, J. (1993) Science for the post-normal age. *Futures*, Vol. 31, n. 7, pp. 735-755.

Funtowicz, S., & Ravetz, J. (1994) Emergent complex systems. *Futures*, Vol. 26, n. 6, pp. 568-582.

Funtowicz, S. (2006) Why knowledge assessment, in Pereira Guimarães Â., Guedes Vas, S, & Tognetti, S. (ed.s) *Interfaces between science and society*. Sheffield: Greenleaf.

Funtowicz, S. (2007) Modelli di scienza e politica, in Modonesi C., Tamino G., Verga I. (ed.s) *Biotecnocrazia: informazione scientifica, agricoltura, decisione politica*. Milano: Jaca Book.

Funtowicz, S., & Strand, R. (2011) Change and commitment: beyond risk and responsibility. *Journal of Risk Research*, Vol.14, pp. 1-9.

Gallopin, G.C., Funtowicz, S., O 'Connor, M., & Ravetz J. (2001) Science for the 21st century: from social contract to the scientific core. *International Journal of Social Science*, Vol. 168, pp. 219-229.

Gausen, D., & Moen, V. (1991) Large-scale escapes of farmed Atlantic salmon (*Salmo salar*) into Norwegian rivers threaten natural populations. *Can. J. Fish. Aquat. Sci.*, Vol. 48, pp. 426–428.

Giampietro, M. (2002), The precautionary principle and ecological hazards of genetically modified organisms, *Ambio*, Vol. 31, n.6, pp. 466-470.

Giampietro M. (1994). Sustainability and technological development in agriculture: a critical appraisal of genetic engineering, *BioScience*, Vol. 44, pp.677-689.

Giampietro, M. (2009) The future of agriculture, in Science for Policy, In: Pereira Guimarães, Â. and Funtowicz, S. (Eds) Oxford: Oxford University Press, pp. 83-104.

Gibbs, W.W. (2003a) The unseen genome: gems among the junk, *Scientific American*, Vol. 289, pp. 46-53, (nov. 2003).

Gibbs, W.W. (2003b) The unseen genome: beyond DNA, *Scientific American*, pp. 108-113, (dec. 2003).

Giovannucci, E., Pollak, M., Liu, Y., Platz, E.A., Majeed, N., Rimm, E.B., & Willett, W.C. (2003) Nutritional predictors of insulin-like growth factor I and their relationships to cancer in men. *Cancer Epidemiology, Biomarkers & Prevention*, Vol. 12, pp. 84-89.

Goldenberg, S. (2011) Obama administration 'bailed out' GM salmon firm. *The Guardian*, October 18, 2011

Grosjean, H., & Benne, R., eds (1998) *Modification and Editing of RNA*. ASM Press, Washington, DC.

Guarnieri, V., Benessia, A., Camino, E., & Barbiero, G. (2008) The myth of natural barriers. Is transgene introgression by GM crops an environmental risk? *Rivista di Biologia - Biology Forum*, Vol. 101, pp. 195-214.

Hardin, S. (2004) Rethinking standpoint epistemology: what is "Strong Objectivity?", in S. Harding (ed.), *The feminist standpoint theory reader: Intellectual and Political Controversies*, London: Routledge, pp. 127-140.

Hedrick, P. W. (2001) Invasion of transgenes from salmon or other genetically modified organisms into natural populations. *Can. J. Fish. Aquat. Sci.*, Vol. 58, pp. 841-844.

Hirotsune, S., Yoshida, N., Chen, A., Garrett, L., Sugiyama, F., Takahashi, S., Yagami, K., Wynshaw-Boris, A., & Yoshiki, A. (2003) An expressed pseudogene regulates the messenger-RNA stability of its homologous coding gene. *Nature*, Vol. 423, pp. 91–96.

Ho, M.W. (1998) *Genetic engineering: Dream or Nightmare?* Continuum International Publishing Group.

Hu, W., & Zhu, Z.Y. (2010) Integration mechanisms of transgenes and population fitness of GH transgenic fish. *Science China - Life Sciences, Vol.* 53, pp. 401-408.

Ibrahim, Y.M. (1996) Genetic soybeans alarm Europeans. *The New York Times,* November 7, 1996.

International Human Genome Sequencing Consortium [IHGSC] (2001) Initial sequencing and analysis of the human genome, *Nature,* Vol. 409, pp. 860-921.

James, C. (2010) *Global Status of Commercialized Biotech/GM Crops: 2010.* ISAAA Brief n. 42. ISAAA: Ithaca, NY.

Jasanoff, S. (1990). *The fifth branch: science advisers and policymakers,* Cambridge Massachusetts: Harvard University Press.

Jasanoff, S. (2003) Technologies of humility: citizen participation in governing science. *Minerva,* Vol. 41, n. 3, pp. 223-244.

Jasanoff, S. (2005) *Designs on nature.* Princeton CA: Princeton University Press.

Jasanoff, S. (2007) Technologies of humility. *Nature,* Vol. 450, p. 33.

Jukes, T.H., & Osawa, S. (1990) The genetic code in mitochondria and chloroplasts. *Experientia,* Vol. 46, n. 11–12, pp. 1117–1126.

Kaplinsky, N., Braun, D., Lish, D., Hay, A., Hake, S., & Freeling, M. (2002) Maize transgene results in Mexico are artefacts. *Nature,* Vol. 416, p. 601.

Kastenhofer, K. (2007) Converging epistemic cultures? A discussion drawing on empirical findings. *Innovation: The European Journal of Social Science Research,* Vol. 20, pp. 359-73.

Kastenhofer, K. (2011) Risk assessment technologies and post-normal science, *Science and Technology for Human Value,* Vol. 36, n. 3, pp. 307-333.

Knorr Cetina, K. (1999) *Epistemic cultures: how the sciences make knowledge.* Cambridge MA: Harvard University Press.

Kuzma, J., & Besley, J. (2008) Ethics of risk analysis and regulatory review: from bio- to nanotechnology. *Nanoethics,* Vol. 2, n. 2, pp. 149-162.

Leggat, L.A., Brauner, C.J., Iwama G.K., & Devlin, R.H. (2007) The glutathione antioxidant system is enhanced in growth hormone transgenic coho salmon (*Oncorhynchus kisutch*). *J. Comparative . Phisiology B: Biochemical, Systemic, and Environmental Physiology,* . Vol. 177, pp. 413-422.

Leptowski, W. (2002) Biotech ok corral. *Science and Policy Perspectives.* Vol. 13. 11.11.2011. Available from: http://www.cspo.org/_old_ourlibrary/documents/060902.html

Lewenstein, B. (2005) What counts as a 'social and ethical issue' in nanotechnology? *HYLE, International Journal for Philosophy of Chemistry,* Vol. 11, n. 1, pp. 5-18.

Liberatore, A., & Funtowicz, S. (2003) 'Democratising' expertise, 'expertising' democracy: what does this mean, and why bother. *Science and public policy,* Vol. 30, n. 3, pp. 146-150.

Losey, J.E., Rayor, L.S., & Carter, M.E. (1999) Transgenic pollen harms monarch larvae. *Nature,* Vol. 399, p. 214.

Lu, Y., Wu, K., Jiang, Y., Xia, B., Li, P., Feng, H., Wyckhuys, K.A.G., & Guo, Y. (2010) Mirid bug outbreaks in multiple crops correlated with wide-scale adoption of Bt cotton in China. *Science,* Vol. 328, pp. 1151-1152.

Mattera, P. (2004). USDA Inc.: How Agribusiness has hijacked regulatory policy at the US Department of Agriculture. Released at the Food and Agriculture Conference of The Organization for Competitive Markets, July 23.Omaha, Nebraska. 9.11.2011. Available from: http://www.nffc.net/Issues/Corporate%20Control/USDA%20INC.pdf

Margulis, L. (1998) *Symbiotic Planet*, Basic Books, New York.

Matlin, A.J., Clark, F., & Smith, C.W.J. (2005). Understanding alternative splicing: towards a cellular code. *Nature Reviews* Vol.6, No.5, pp. 386–398.

McClintock, B. (1950) The origin and behavior of mutable loci in maize. *Proc Natl Acad Sci USA*, Vol.36, No.6, pp. 344–355.

McKinnell, S., Thomson, A.J., Black, E.A., Wing, B.L., Guthrie III, C.M., Koerner, J.F., & Helle, J.H. (1997). Atlantic salmon in the North Pacific. *Aquacult. Res.*, Vol. 28, pp. 145–157.

McLaren, J.S. (2005) Crop biotechnology provides an opportunity to develop a sustainable future. *Trends in Biotechnology*, Vol. 23, n. 7, pp. 339–342.

Meghani, Z. (2009) The FDA, normativity of risk assessment, GMOs, and the American democracy. *Journal of Agriculture and Environmental Ethics*, Vol. 22, pp. 125-139.

Meghani, Z., & Kuzma, J. (2011) The "revolving door" between regulatory agencies and industry: a problem that requires reconceptualizing objectivity. *Journal of Agriculture and Environmental Ehtics*, Vol. 24, pp. 575-599.

Metz, M., & Fütterer, J. (2002) Suspect evidence of transgenic contamination. *Nature*, Vol. 416, pp. 600-601.

Mighell, A.J., Smith, N.R., Robinson, P.A., & Markham, A.F. (2000) Vertebrate pseudogenes. *FEBS Lett.*, Vol. 468, n. .2–3, pp. 109–114.

Monbiot, G. (2002) The fake persuaders: corporations are inventing people to rubbish their opponents on the Internet. *The Guardian*, May 14, 2002.

Muir, W. M., & Howard, R.D. (1999) Possible ecological risks of transgenic organism release when transgenes affect mating success: sexual selection and the Trojan gene hypothesis. *Proc. Natl. Acad. Sci. USA*, Vol. 96, pp. 13853-13856.

Neumann, W., & Pollack, A. (2010) Farmers cope with roundup-resistant weeds. *The New York Times*, May 3, 2010.

Nuffield Bioethics Committee (2004) The Use of Genetically Modified Crops in Developing Countries. 8.11.2011. Available from: http://www.nuffieldbioethics.org/gm-crops-developing-countries

Organisation for Economic Co-operation and Development (1993) *Safety Evaluation of Foods Derived by Modern Biotechnology: 'Concepts and Principles'*. 9.11.2011. Available from: http://dbtbiosafety.nic.in/guideline/OACD/Concepts_and_Principles_1993.pdf

Perrow, C. (1984) *Normal accidents: living with high risks technologies*. New York: Basic Books.

Piñeyro-Nelson, A., Van Heerwaarden, J., Perales, H.R., Serratos-Hernández, J.A., Rangel, A., Hufford, M.B., Gepts, P., Garay-Arroyo, A., Rivera-Bustamante, R., & Álvarez-Buylla, E. R. (2009) Transgenes in Mexican maize: molecular evidence and methodological considerations for GMO detection in landrace populations. *Molecular Ecology*, Vol. 18, n. 4, pp. 750-761.

Pollack, A. (2007) Without U.S. Rules, Biotech food lacks investors, *The New York Times*, July 30.

Pollan, M. (2001) The Great Yellow Hype, *The New York Times Magazine*, March 4, 2001.

Potrykus, I. (2010) Regulations must be revolutionized. *Nature*, Vol. 466, p. 561.

Poliseno, L., Salmena, L., Zhang, J., Carver, B, Haveman, W.J., & Pandolfi, P.P. (2010) A coding-independent function of gene and pseudogene mRNAs regulates tumour biology. *Nature*, Vol. 465, pp. 1033–1038.

Prigogine, I. (1978) *From being to becoming*, San Francisco, Ca.: W.H. Freeman and Company.

Princeton University (2009) 'Junk' DNA has important role, researchers find. *ScienceDaily*. 11.07.2010. Available from:
www.sciencedaily.com/releases/2009/05/090520140408.htm

Pring, D., Brennicke, A., & Schuster, W. (1993) RNA editing gives a new meaning to the genetic information in mitochondria and chloroplasts. *Plant Mol. Biol.*, Vol. 21, n. 6, pp. 1163–1170.

Quist, D., & Chapela, I. H. (2001) Transgenic DNA introgressed into traditional maize landraces in Oaxaca, Mexico. *Nature*, Vol. 414, pp. 541-543.

Quist, D., & Chapela, I. H. (2002) Quist and Chapela reply. *Nature*, Vol. 416, p. 602.

Ravetz, J. (2001) Safety in the globalizing knowledge economy: an analysis by paradoxes, *J Hazard Mater.*, Vol. 86, n. 1-3, pp. 1-16.

Ravetz, J. (2003) A paradoxical future for safety in the global knowledge economy, *Futures*, Vol. 35, n. 8, pp. 811-826.

Ravetz, J. (2004) The post-normal science of precaution. *Futures*, Vol. 36, n. 3, pp. 347-357.

Revolving Door Working Group - RDWG (2005). *A matter of trust: how the revolving door undermines public confidence in government and what to do about it. Journal of Agriculture Environmental Ethics*, Vol.24, pp. 575-579.

Roberts, S.B., McCauley, L.A.R., Devlin, R.H., & Goetz, F.W. (2004) Transgenic salmon overexpressing growth hormone exhibit decreased myostatin transcript and protein expression. *Journal of Experimental Biology*, Vol. 207, pp. 3741-3748.

Rockström, J., Steffen, W., Noone, N., Persson, Å., Chapin, F.S. III, Lambin, E.F., Lenton, T.M., Scheffer, M., Folke, C., Schellnhuber, H.J., Nykvist, B., de Wit, C.A., Hughes, T., van der Leeuw, S., Rodhe, H., Sörlin, S., Snyder, P.K., Costanza, R., Svedin, U., Falkenmark, M., Karlberg, L., Corell, R.W., Fabry, V.J., Hansen, J., Walzer, B., Liverman, D., Richardson, K., Crutzen, P., & Foley, J.A. (2009) A safe operating space for humanity. *Nature*, Vol. 461, 472-475.

Saenz, A. (2010) Genetically Engineered 'EnviroPig' Waiting For US Approval. 7.11.2011. Available from: http://singularityhub.com

Sarewitz, D. (2004) How science makes environmental controversies worse. *Environmental science and policy*, Vol. 7, pp. 385-403.

Sarewitz, D. (2011) The voice of science: let's agree to disagree. *Nature*, Vol. 478, p. 7.

Shapiro, J. A. (2009) Revisiting the central dogma in the 21st century. *Ann. N Y Acad. Sci.*, Vol. 1178, pp. 6–28.

Shiva, V. (1997) *Biopiracy. The plunder of nature and knowledge*. Cambridge MA: South End Press.

Shrader-Frechette, K.S. (1996) Methodological rules for four classes of scientific uncertainty. In Lemons, J. (eds.) *Scientific Uncertainty and Environmental Problem Solving*. Oxford: Blackwell.

Siomi, H., & Siomi, M. C. (2009) On the road to reading the RNA-interference code. *Nature*, Vol. 457, pp. 396–404.

Skalka, M.A., & Goff, S.P. (1993) *Reverse transcriptase* (1st ed.). New York: Cold Spring Harbor.

Smith M.D., Asche F., Guttormsen A.G., & Wiener J.B. (2010). Genetically Modified Salmon and Full Impact Assessment. *Science*, Vol. 330, n. 6007, pp. 1052-1053.

Smith, R., & Wynne, B. (1989) *Expert evidence: interpreting science in the law*. London: Routledge.

Snow, A. (2009) Unwanted transgenes re-discovered in Oaxacan Maize. *Molecular Ecology*, Vol. 18, n. 4 , pp. 569-571.

Stewart, N.C. Jr., Halfhill, D.M., & Warwick, S.I. (2003) Transgene introgression from genetically modified crops to their wild relatives. *Nature Reviews Genetic*, Vol. 4, pp. 806-817.

Stewart, N.C. Jr. (2004) *Genetically modified planet: environmental impacts of genetically modified plants*. Oxford: Oxford University Press.

Storz, G. (2002) An expanding universe of noncoding RNAs. *Science*, Vol. 296, pp. 1260-1263.

Sundström, L.F., Lohmus, M., Johnsson, J.I., & Devlin, R.H. (2004) Growth hormone transgenic salmon pay for growth potential with increased predation mortality. *Proceedings of the Royal Society of London. Series B, Biological Sciences*. Vol. 271, Suppl. 5, pp. S350-S352.

Sundström, L.F., Lohmus, M., Tymchuk, W.E,. & Devlin, R.H. (2007). Gene–environment interactions influence ecological consequences of transgenic animals. *Proc. Natl. Acad. Sci. USA*, Vol. 104, pp. 3889-3894.

Tallacchini, M.C. (2005) Before and beyond the precautionary principle: epistemology of uncertainty in science and law. *Toxicology and applied pharmacology*, Vol. 207, pp. 645-651.

Tallacchini, M.C. (2000) Lo stato epistemico: la regolazione giuridica della scienza, in Mazzani C. (ed.) *Etica della ricerca biologica*. Firenze: Olschki.

Temin, H.M., & Mizutani, S. (1970) Viral RNA-dependent DNA Polymerase: RNA-dependent DNA Polymerase in virions of Rous Sarcoma Virus. *Nature*, Vol. 226, pp. 1211-1213.

Time Magazine (2000) July 31, Vol. 156, n.5.

Townsend, A. R., & Howarth, R. W. (2010) Fixing the global Nitrogen problem, *Scientific American*, October, pp. 64-71.

Travis, J. (2002) Biological dark matter. *Science News Online*, Jan. 12, 2002. 14.04.2011. Available from: www.sciencenews.org/articles/20020112/bob9.asp

Tucker, B.J. & Breaker, R.R. (2005) Riboswitches as versatile gene control elements. *Curr Opin Struct Biol*, Vol. 15, n. 3, pp. 342–348.

Union of Concerned Scientists (2009) Failure to yield: Evaluating the performance of genetically modified yields. 8.11.2011. Available from: www.ucsusa.org/assets/documents/food_and_agriculture/failure-to-yield.pdf

U.S. Food and Drug Administration (2009) Genetically Engineered Animals Diagram. In Final Guidance on Regulating Genetically Engineered Animals. 28.10.2011. Available from: http://www.fda.gov/ForConsumers/ConsumerUpdates/ucm143980.htm

U.S. Food and Drug Administration Center for Veterinary Medicine (2009) Guidance for industry: *Regulation of genetically engineered animals containing heritable recombinant DNA constructs*. 19.09.2011. Available from:

http://www.fda.gov/downloads/AnimalVeterinary/GuidanceComplianceEnforc
ement/GuidanceforIndustry/UCM113903.pdf

U.S. Food and Drug Administration Center for Veterinary Medicine - Veterinary Medicine Advisory Committee (2010) *Briefing Packet* AquAdvantage salmon. 11.06.2011. Available from:
http://www.fda.gov/downloads/AdvisoryCommittees/CommitteesMeetingMate
rials/VeterinaryMedicineAdvisoryCommittee/UCM224762.pdf

Vassallo, P., Bastianoni, S., Beiso, I, Ridolfi, R., & Fabiano M. (2007) Emergy analysis for the environmental sustainability of an inshore fish farming system. Ecological Indicators, Vol. 7, pp. 290–298.

Venter, J.C., *et al. ii* 274 authors (2001) The sequence of the human genome. *Science*, Vol. 291, pp. 1304-1351.

Vitreschak, A.G., Rodionov, D.A., Mironov, A.A., & Gelfand, M.S. (2004) Riboswitches: the oldest mechanism for the regulation of gene expression? *Trends Genet*, Vol. 20, n. 1, pp. 44–50.

Waltner-Toews, D., & Lang, T. (2000) A new conceptual base for food and agricultural policy: The emerging model of links between agriculture, food, health, environment and society. *Global Change and Human Health*, Vol. 1, n. 2, pp. 116-130.

Weinberg, A.M. (1972) Science and transcience, *Minerva*, Vol. 10, pp. 209-222.

Wicker, T., Sabot, F., Hua-Van, A., Bennetzen, J.L., Capy, P., Chalhoub, B., Flavell, A., Leroy, P., Morgante, M., Panaud, O., Paux, E., SanMiguel, P., & Schulman, A.H. (2007) A unified classification system for eukaryotic transposable elements. *Nature Reviews Genetics*, Vol. 8, n .12, pp. 973–982.

Wildavsky, A. (1979) *Speaking truth to power*. Boston: Little Brown and Co.

Wynne, B., Felt, U., Callon, M., Gonçalves, M.E., Jasanoff, S., Jepsen, M., Joly, P.B., Konopasek, Z, May, S., Naeubauer, C., Arie, R., Siune, K., Stirlig, A., & Tallacchini, M.C. (2007) *Taking Knowledge Society Seriously. European Commission*: EUR 22700 EN.

Yaskowiak, E.S., Shears, M.A., Agarwal-Mawal, A., & Fletcher, G.L. (2006) Characterization and multi-generational stability of the growth hormone transgene (EO-1α) responsible for enhanced growth rates in Atlantic salmon. *Transgenic Research, Vol.* 15, pp. 465-480.

Zangerl, A.R., McKenna, D., Wraight, C.L., Carroll, M., Ficarello, P., Warner, R., & Berenbaum, M.R. (2001) Effects of exposure to event 176 *Bacillus thuringiensis* corn pollen on monarch and black swallowtail caterpillars under field conditions. *Proceedings of the National Academy of Sciences*, Vol. 98, pp. 11908-11912.

Ziman, J. (1984) *An introduction to science studies*, Cambridge, UK: Cambridge University Press.

5

Xenotropic Murine Leukemia Virus-Related Virus as a Case Study: Using a Precautionary Risk Management Approach for Emerging Blood-Borne Pathogens in Canada

Michael G. Tyshenko et al.*
McLaughlin Centre for Population Health Risk Assessment, Institute of Population Health, University of Ottawa, Ontario, Canada

1. Introduction

In October 2009 it was reported that 68 of 101 patients with chronic fatigue syndrome (CFS) in the United States, when tested, were infected with a novel gamma retrovirus, xenotropic murine leukemia virus-related virus (XMRV) (Lombardi et al., 2009). XMRV is a recently discovered human gammaretrovirus first described in prostate cancers that shares significant homology with murine leukemia virus (MLV) (Ursiman et al., 2006). It is known that XMRV can cause leukemias and sarcomas in several rodent, feline, and primate species but has not been shown to cause disease in humans. XMRV was detectable in the peripheral blood mononuclear cells (PBMCs) and plasma of individuals diagnosed with CFS (Lombardi et al., 2009). After this report was published there was a great deal of uncertainty surrounding this emergent virus and its involvement in the etiology of CFS. The uncertainty was, in part, due to CFS being a complex, poorly understood multi-system disorder with different disease criteria used for its diagnosis. CFS, also known as Myalgic Encephalomyelitis (ME), is a debilitating disease of unknown origin that is estimated to affect 17 million people worldwide. The initial report connecting XMRV to prostate cancers and CFS garnered significant media and scientific interest since it provided a potential

* Susie ElSaadany[2]**, Tamer Oraby[1], Marian Laderoute[2], Jun Wu[2], Willy Aspinall[3],
Daniel Krewski[1, 4] and Peter R. Ganz[5]
[1]*McLaughlin Centre for Population Health Risk Assessment, Institute of Population Health, University of Ottawa, Ontario, Canada*
[2]*Blood Safety Surveillance and Health Care Acquired Infections Division, Centre for Communicable Diseases and Infection Control, Public Health Agency of Canada, Ottawa, Ontario, Canada*
[3]*Aspinall and Associates, Cleveland House, High Street, and Earth Sciences, Bristol University, Bristol, United Kingdom*
[4]*Department of Epidemiology and Community Medicine, Faculty of Medicine, University of Ottawa, Ottawa, Ontario, Canada*
[5]*Health Canada, Director's Office, Ottawa, Ontario, Canada*
** Corresponding Author

explanation for the disease but also an avenue for possible therapeutic treatments since XMRV is known to be susceptible to some anti-retroviral drugs (Cohen, 2011).

The results first reported by Lombardi et al. (2009) suggested that there may be a strong relationship between XMRV infections and CFS. However, other studies later completed from North America (Switzer et al., 2010), Europe (Groom et al., 2010; van Kuppeveld et al., 2010) and China (Hong et al., 2010) failed to find any XMRV associated with CFS patient samples.

Since XMRV was putatively associated with CFS (Lombardi et. al, 2009) and prostate cancer patient groups (Urisman et al., 2006; Schlaberg et al., 2009), these patient groups' blood policies as donor groups were of greatest concern. Individuals previously diagnosed with cancer are already deferred in Canada[1], so the main issue of the need for new policy focused squarely on XMRV and its linkage with CFS. Data from the 2002-2003 Canadian Community Health Survey revealed that about 5% of those surveyed self-reported as having been diagnosed with at least one of the following conditions: CFS, fibromyalgia or multiple chemical sensitivity. Extrapolating from this study it is estimated that approximately 341,000 Canadians self-reported as being diagnosed with CFS. If a confirmed linkage between XMRV and CFS was established this would have a significant impact on policies for blood safety, as well as cells, tissues and organ (CTO) transplantation.

Other retroviruses such as human immunodeficiency virus (HIV) and human T-lymphotropic virus (HTLV) have been shown to infect human cell lines and lymphocytes when the virus is taken from human samples; also these retroviruses are known to be transmitted by transfusion (Lombardi et al., 2009). MLV-like virus was reported in symptomatic patients persisting for over a decade and the detection of XMRV in healthy controls suggested that asymptomatic carriers also likely existed within the donor population (Lo et al., 2010; Lombardi et al., 2009). These research studies highlighted that XMRV could be a potential emerging threat to transfusion/transplantation of blood, cells, tissues and organ safety globally.

Uncertainty over XMRV as an emerging blood-borne pathogen was confounded by considerable information gaps in the available peer review literature. The lack of published research studies in this area was confirmed by a PubMED[2] database search conducted June 1, 2010 using the keywords "XMRV" which resulted in a scant number of 43 peer reviewed papers beginning from the year 2006 when the first paper on this topic was published. The search results highlight how recent this topic area was for researchers and decision-makers alike. Moreover, it reflected how little research and scientific information was available to help inform evidence-based decision making.

By late 2011 the situation surrounding XMRV and its uncertainty as a new emerging pathogen appeared to be largely resolved. Several published scientific studies indicated that XMRV positives reported in previously published cohort studies were likely the result of contamination (Hue et al., 2010; Kaiser, 2011; Carlowe 2011; Smith, 2010). In October 2011

---

[1] Permanently if they are blood donors, and for five years if they are cell tissue or organ (CTO) donors; they can be CTO donors only if there is no evidence of disease return.
[2] NCBI PubMED: http://www.ncbi.nlm.nih.gov/entrez/query.fcgi?db=PubMed. PubMED includes over 15 million peer review citations of scientific research articles from the 1950s to present day.

the co-authors of the original research paper published in 2009 that described detection of XMRV in blood cells of patients with CFS (as reported in Lombardi et al., 2009) issued a partial retraction. A re-examination of the samples used showed that some of the CFS PBMC DNA preparations were contaminated with XMRV plasmid DNA (Silverman et al., 2011). The idea of mouse DNA contamination in some laboratories and reagents provides the most parsimonious explanation for the geographic differences found in patient cohort studies completed in different countries and the inability to reproduce XMRV positives.

Sample contamination appeared to stem from multiple sources. In one study, Robinson et al. (2010) analyzed mouse DNA contamination in human tissue samples and also tested for XMRV. The results showed that contamination with mouse DNA was widespread in formalin fixed paraffin embedded human prostate tissue samples detectable by polymerase chain reaction (PCR) assays that targeted a high copy number mouse DNA sequence (intracisternal A particle long terminal repeat DNA). It was also reported by several research laboratories that an endogenous murine leukemia viral genome contaminant was found in a commercial reverse transcriptase-polymerase chain reaction (RT-PCR) kit used in some studies to detect XMRV. In some cases, the PCR "master mixes" used contained small amounts of contaminating mouse DNA sequences that were amplified during testing of human samples. Amplification occurred due to the high degree of sequence similarity between the XRMV oligonucleotide primers used and the contaminating mouse nucleic acids (Bacich et al., 2011; Sato et al., 2010; Tuke et al., 2010; Oakes et al., 2010; Knox et al., 2011).

A re-evaluation of blood samples from 61 patients with CFS by PCR and RT-PCR methods for the detection of viral nucleic acids and assays used to detect infectious virus and virus-specific antibodies revealed no evidence of XMRV. Initially, 43 of these samples had tested positive for XMRV. The results were consistent with previous reports that detected MLV nucleic acid sequences in commercial reagents and that the previous evidence linking XMRV and MLVs to CFS was likely attributable to contamination (Knox et al., 2011).

Other follow-on studies confirmed that XMRV appeared to be a contaminant of prostate cells lines and human tissue samples. Investigation into an existing permanent prostate cell line, 22Rv1 which is widely used as it is one of very few cell lines available to study androgen-independent prostate cancer, revealed that prior to 1996, the cell line did not contain XMRV DNA. The authors suggested the presence of XMRV after this time was likely an introduced artifact (Cohen, 2011; Yang et al., 2011). Moreover, further investigation revealed that XMRV was not present in the original CWR22 tumor used to generate the prostate cell line but it arose by recombination of two overlapping and highly homologous proviruses (PreXMRV-1 and PreXMRV-2) that were present in the mice during tumor passaging. Paprotka et al. (2011) proposed that the association of XMRV with human disease was due to contamination of human samples with virus originating from this recombination event. However, it did not explain earlier outbreaks of CFS-ME which occurred prior to 1996 nor that some of the patients who tested positive for XMRV had disease onset prior to 1996.

Thus, the early differences reported in peer review literature during the 2009 to 2010 time period and the eventual resolution surrounding XMRV as a contamination artifact by mid-2011 provide an interesting case study to review for the application of precautionary action when managing emerging blood-borne pathogens. The question of "when to act and exercise precaution" given an emerging threat to blood safety with high uncertainty is important for ensuring public health safety for blood transfusions and transplantation of CTOs.

2. Expert discussion for XMRV as an emerging blood-borne pathogen

The 2009-2010 time period presented a significant challenge to health policy requiring management decisions for XMRV as a potential emerging threat to blood and CTO safety. The context was of a lack of available risk information, a lack of an approved diagnostic test for large-scale blood screening, a virus with a relatively high prevalence rate in the general population and defined patient groups (eg., CFS cohorts and prostate cancer groups, as reported by a limited number of research studies), and contradictory research results from different patient clinical samples estimation of XMRV prevalence (e.g., North American versus European XMRV clinical studies). Early risk management decisions must be based on data which is scarce, for a risk that is emerging, highly uncertain and largely unquantified.

In Canada, one of the early risk management steps was to convene a group of experts to discuss the risks associated with XMRV. To address this uncertainty and to inform decision making as a tool to guide public health policy, a half-day workshop was held to discuss the issues and relevant questions about XMRV knowledge gaps. The "International Risk Assessment Workshop Results for XMRV with respect to Blood, Cells, Tissues and Organ Safety Structured Expert Elicitation" policy workshop was held on September 29, 2010 in Ottawa, Canada. The focus was to discuss various XMRV issues within a policy and risk management context.

Experts discussed various related issues including: scientific uncertainty and contradictory XMRV data reported in peer review literature; the prevalence of XMRV; risk parameters affecting XMRV transmission; latency of XMRV; routes of XMRV transmission; risk mitigation of XMRV (the use of leukoreduction); and XMRV disease relationships (whether or not the virus causal or non-causal for CFS, prostate cancer or other diseases).

Expert opinion can be used to address such questions and provide insight into the uncertainties surrounding emerging risks where scientific data is missing, sparse or uninformative. Expert opinion can, at the very least, provide useful indications of possible risks and a robust discussion of pertinent issues for which current data preclude a direct evidence-based assessment (Aspinall, 2010). Such indications can, in turn, inform risk management decision making about emerging risks which must be made even in the face of significant uncertainty. In the absence of more definitive data, expert elicitation can be used to inform policy responses to emerging threats as they occur, and help prioritize issues until scientific research is in a position to support evidenced-based risk management policy development.

3. Scientific uncertainty and contradictory XMRV data

During the expert workshop a number of plausible reasons were postulated to explain the variability in XMRV prevalence data reported in different countries.[3] First, there may be

---

[3] Note that during the time of the workshop (September, 2010) there were no published research studies confirming mouse DNA contamination of patient samples or contamination of diagnostic test kits with minute quantities of mouse genetic material that could result in XMRV false positives.

greater sequence diversity in XMRV variants than originally observed. As a result, PCR oligonucleotide primers with mismatches used in different studies may not amplify XMRV sequence variants as effectively, resulting in missed positive samples.

Second, *in vivo* reservoir(s) of viral replication may not identified suggesting that other tissues may be better for testing than PBMCs. Cells, other than leukocytes, may be the primary target cell infected *in vivo*. Until 2010, most negative XMRV studies used DNA prepared from PBMCs for PCR testing but XMRV virus may be present predominantly as plasma viremia which would be difficult to detect if only these cells were analysed by PCR.

Third, XMRV sequence within the population may be more heterologous than the known published sequences. All negative studies tested for the virus using only the VP62 prototypical prostate XMRV strain sequences. Lombardi et al. (2009) in their study showed XMRV in a high percentage of CFS patients using culture and serology in addition to PCR testing. At the time the experts cautioned that until more was known about viral reservoirs for XMRV, the replication rates and the viral sequence diversity that the use of a single stand-alone assay (such as real time and single round PCR on fresh patient materials) may not be enough to detect true positive cases.

Fourth, the worldwide distribution of XMRV is low and scattered like HTLV-1 making its detection in clinical patient groups difficult to confirm. The low viral load in conjunction with the test procedures used, including the sample's preparation, treatment and storage varied between the different studies which could have affected XMRV detection.

Fifth, patient selection and methods applied to different studies varied widely; this could result in samples from patients who are not true CFS cases. Differences in the patient groups studied that were from different geographic areas and the variability in patients within these groups for CFS disease severity and duration may have affected results. There were and are variations in the different CFS case definitions in use. For example, the most widely used CFS case definition is the Fukuda, USA CDC criteria (Fukuda et al., 1994). Other CFS case definitions used to select research subjects include the Canadian Consensus Criteria for CFS-ME published in 2003 (Carruthers et al., 2003), Holmes et al.'s CFS working case definition (Holmes et al., 1988), the Oxford criteria (Sharpe et al., 1991) and the CDC clinically empirical approach (Reeves et al., 2005).

In hindsight, the variability in XMRV detection was likely due to mouse DNA or VP62 plasmid contamination within samples and/or the use of mouse DNA contaminated RT-PCR kits as later detailed by various studies (Sato et al., 2010; Robinson et al., 2010).

4. Prevalence of XMRV

The experts indicated that estimating an overall worldwide prevalence for XMRV was difficult as differences in regional demographics exist. However, the experts considered the prevalence in the UK, France, USA and Canada to be nearly the same. The experts indicated that there was a clear need for more evidence regarding XMRV incidence, for example completing an age stratified prevalence study or a simple cross-section of prevalence was suggested as a key experiment that would help to inform this answer.

In Canada, the National Microbiology Laboratory (Public Health Agency of Canada, Winnipeg) had undertaken a number of laboratory studies on XMRV, focusing on screening for X/P-MLV related virus sequences in healthy controls and patients with multiple blood transfusions. Groups tested included a small blood bank repository (n = 84), Canadian Blood and Marrow Transplant Group (CBMTG) (n = 54), Canadian Blood Services Registry (n = 76 plasma samples and n = 29 buffy coat samples from hemophiliacs), Canadian Aphaeresis Group - Thrombotic thrombocytopenic purpura patients (n = 23), liver transplant patients (n = 21) and HEV/HCV genotyping samples (n = 94, comprised of 75 HCV and 9 HEV samples). Despite testing a number of at-risk patients and multiply transfused patients with single round PCR methods only 1 patient in the CBMTG group (1.8%) and 3 out of 75 HCV patients (4%) were XMRV positive. All of the other samples showed no evidence of XMRV by nucleic acid testing (Dr. Anton Andonov, Public Health Agency of Canada, personal communication). Results from testing Canadian patients showed little XMRV associated with CFS patient or high risk patient groups.

5. Risk parameters for XMRV

The experts displayed good group agreement on the median age of infection for XMRV of approximately 26 years with a range from 2 to 63 years. The experts believed that the proportion of men to women was 1:1 regarding XMRV infectivity; in other words, the experts did not think that there was a gender bias for XMRV infection within human populations. Position R462Q in the ribonuclease L (RNAse L) protein is known to be an important factor for antiviral response activation. This single nucleotide polymorphism (SNP) in RNAse L has been shown to block viral replication by degrading single stranded viral RNA and it is strongly implicated in the prevention of infection *in vivo* (Urisman et al., 2006). However, the experts believed that RNAse L SNP R462Q genetic susceptibility was not an important factor for the relative risk of XMRV infection (eg., being RR, RQ or QQ genotype for RNAse L at position 462 has little impact on infectivity).

Latency of XMRV was also considered to be an important risk factor. The experts believed that not all XMRV infections may result in persistent infections (transient infections may occur) and there was a need for nucleic acid testing detection in blood and plasma to include persistent viremia in chronically infected individuals. Experts believed that the majority of individuals infected with XMRV longer than three months (chronic infections) would have detectable antibodies and have detectable nucleic acids by nucleic acid testing (NAT) of their blood. The experts believed that the vast majority of individuals infected with XMRV were likely asymptomatic.

6. Routes of transmission for XMRV

To assess XMRV transmission the experts were asked to rank the risks associated with 12 potential routes of XMRV transmission using the method of pairwise comparisons (Macutkiewicz, 2008). With this approach, experts were presented with 12C2 = 66 pairs of routes, and asked to indicate which of the two routes being compared they considered to be riskier. In the pairwise comparison exercise, a draft list of XMRV transmission risk routes was presented to the expert group. The list was modified and agreed upon by the experts after discussing the issues involved, and reaching group consensus on the definitions and related information pertinent to each of the transmission routes. The list of 12 potential routes of XMRV transmission is given in Tables 1 and 2.

The expert group's risk rankings associated with XMRV transmission were determined using the Probabilistic Inversion (PI) modeling option in UNIBALANCE (© TU Delft, available from: http://risk2.ewi.tudelft.nl/courses). This method produces a mean score for each of the transmission routes rated by the experts, with the standard deviation of the mean score providing a measure of uncertainty in expert opinion. The mean scores are rescaled to be between zero and one, so that the highest score is one (representing the route of transmission seen as most risky by the experts) and the lowest score is zero (the least risky transmission route).

The method is sophisticated enough to allow for both ties in ranking individual pairs of transmission routes being compared and inconsistencies in rankings across risk pairs. In addition to producing an overall ranking of the routes of transmission, the method provides a statistical test of the null hypothesis that a given expert is responding at random (in which case the results for that expert would be excluded from the analysis). The method also provides a test for inconsistency in response for a given expert. Finally, an overall coefficient of agreement ranging between 0 (complete disagreement) and 1 (complete agreement) among the experts is produced. Tests of inconsistency demonstrated that one of the experts appeared to give pairwise preferences randomly; this expert's responses were filtered out leaving 13 experts for the analysis.[4]

The unnormalized mean scores and associated standard deviations for the 12 potential routes of transmission of XMRV are given in Table 1. The normalized scores, anchored at zero (lowest perceived risk) and one (highest perceived risk), are shown in Table 2.

Rank	Transmission Route	Score	Standard deviation
1	Non-leukoreduced packed red blood cells	0.6982	0.2344
2	Solid organs	0.6915	0.2654
3	Bone marrow transplant	0.6655	0.2057
4	Hematopoietic stem cell transplant	0.6329	0.2454
5	Plasma transfusion	0.6113	0.2409
6	Leukoreduced packed red blood cells	0.5036	0.2488
7	Semen	0.4966	0.2537
8	Islet cells	0.3742	0.1963
9	Human derived urinary products	0.3431	0.2109
10	Tissues	0.2593	0.1885
11	Plasma derived clotting factor	0.2043	0.1926
12	Albumin	0.1991	0.1685

Table 1. Results of the pairwise comparison exercise unnormalized scores and standard deviation for 12 different XMRV transmission routes are shown.

---

[4] For more information and summary of the mathematical method used see, "Appendix 2. Description of the pairwise comparison by probabilistic inversion method" in: Tyshenko et al., (2011). For more information about the numerical algorithms used in this method see Macutkiewicz (2008).

The normalized scores indicate that, in relative terms, the ranking of the 12 routes from the most risky route to the least risky route were: non-leukoreduced packed red blood cells, solid organs, bone marrow transplant, hematopoietic stem cell transplant, plasma transfusion, leukoreduced packed red blood cells, semen, islet cells, human derived urinary products, tissue transplants, plasma derived clotting factor and albumin. Even though non-leukoreduced packed red blood cells were ranked as the highest risk the top four risks of non-leukoreduced packed RBC, solid organs, bone marrow transplant and hematopoietic stem cell transplants showed a non-significant difference. The four lowest perceived risks of XMRV transmission were human derived urinary products, tissues, plasma derived clotting factors and albumin. The lower values reflected the experts' views that processing clearance factors and product treatments likely reduce XMRV. Tissue was cited as being a low risk due to the lack of vasculature which would carry much less risk as compared to blood or solid organs. Experts believed albumin also possessed the smallest standard deviation which can be interpreted as having the least uncertainty in its ranking.

Relative Ranking	Transmission Route	Score (normalized)
1	Non-leukoreduced packed RBC	1
2	Solid organs	0.9867
3	Bone marrow transplant	0.9344
4	Hematopoietic stem cell transplant	0.8691
5	Plasma transfusion	0.8259
6	Leukoreduced packed RBC	0.6102
7	Semen	0.5962
8	Islet cells	0.3508
9	Human derived urinary products	0.2885
10	Tissue	0.1206
11	Plasma derived clotting factor	0.0104
12	Albumin	0

Table 2. Results of the pairwise comparison exercise showing the group's normalized scores ranked between 0 and 1 according to relative risk for 12 different XMRV transmission routes.

Overall, the experts considered 12 different routes of transmission, and all were deemed to be either medium to low for their probability to transmit XMRV infectivity. Transmission through blood and blood products split experts into two groups reflecting the uncertainty of XMRV virus infection as to whether it was cell or plasma based. Experts indicated the number of copies of virus in plasma could be variable depending on which stage of infection the donor is at. Regardless, the experts believed non-leukoreduced packed red blood cells, solid organs (due to their vasculature), bone marrow transplants, hematopoietic stem cell transplants, plasma transfusion and leukoreduced packed red blood cells would present the most likely transmission routes for XMRV (> 0.5). Other routes (< 0.5) including: semen, islet cells, human derived urinary products, plasma derived clotting factor, tissues and albumin would be the least likely to transmit XMRV given the list presented.

Xenotropic Murine Leukemia Virus-Related Virus as a Case Study: Using a Precautionary Risk Management
Approach for Emerging Blood-Borne Pathogens in Canada

101

Experts ascribed low values to urine-derived pharmaceuticals (donor pool contaminated by 1 positive individual) due to low numbers of viral particles, large batches (10,000 in a donor pool) and clearance factor during purification. Experts discussed other routes of XMRV transmission not given on the pairwise comparison list and agreed transmission through breast milk and *in vitro* fertilization (IVF) techniques would be low. Similarly, fluids and cells free of white blood cells or plasma were also deemed to be low risk for XMRV transmission. Organs were seen as being riskier than tissues due to vascular systems and immunosuppression of the host. The individual discussions of other XMRV transmission routes correlated well with the results of the more structured pairwise comparison exercise that the expert group completed.

7. Risk mitigation of XMRV

Previous examples of Health Canada's regulatory actions based on a precautionary approach included actions to mitigate the risk of variant Creutzfeldt-Jakob disease (vCJD) and simian foamy virus (SFV) transmission. In both cases donor screening was added to defer those individuals with the highest exposure risk. For vCJD those with travel or residency history in high risk areas (United Kingdom and France) were deferred. The deferral took into account effects on the blood supply balanced against maximal risk reduction. As a result, the risk to transfusion recipients for vCJD was greatly reduced (Wilson et al., 2003). Similarly, donor screening for individuals at risk of exposure to SFV was implemented. Donor demographic screens balanced maximal risk reduction against the impacts to the blood supply. The risk of introduction of a retrovirus with the possibility of developing pathogenicity over time with spread in human hosts by transfusion has been reduced by precautionary actions.[5]

Considering XMRV, there were several risk mitigation options under consideration including: 1) Keeping the status quo, with further research, 2) Education and self-deferral, 3) Deferring donors presumed at risk for carrying XMRV, 4) Testing of donors for XMRV (not currently possible at the time of the expert meeting), and 5) Pathogen reduction strategies (a possible strategy for some components).

In Canada as of March 2010, individuals donating blood at Canadian Blood Services with a diagnosis of CFS were indefinitely deferred from blood donation. Prostate cancer patients are permanently deferred from blood donation, and donations from individuals, who were diagnosed with cancer post-donation, are retrieved, quarantined and destroyed.

Leukoreduction has been a useful risk mitigation strategy applied to other blood-borne pathogens. A Directive on Universal Leukoreduction was issued by Health Canada in 1998 specifying that in Canada that all cellular blood components must be filtered to remove white blood cells (WBCs) and residual WBC levels must be less than 5×10^6 cells per component (Health Canada, 1998). This action which is already in place in Canada was expected to have some protective effect for XMRV knowing that it was mostly associated with WBCs. Further validation studies would be needed to demonstrate the effectiveness of leukoreduction in preventing XMRV transmission through transfusion. The virus could still

---

[5] For donor deferral of SFV in Canada see: http://www.hc-sc.gc.ca/dhp-mps/brgtherap/activit/fs-fi/fact_simian_foamy_virus_spumeux_simien_feuillet-eng.php

be transmitted through plasma but data was lacking concerning titres necessary for infection.

The experts estimated a central value of 3 log reductions by leukoreduction but gave a consensus range that spanned 7 logs suggesting some uncertainty about the degree of clearance. Some experts highlighted the fact that whether the virus was cell-associated or from plasma viremia was an important consideration when determining the effectiveness of leukoreduction since this method likely would not reduce virus load found in plasma. When asked, the experts indicated that they had considered both cell-associated and plasma-associated virus when answering this question.

Experts believed plasma derivatives would have higher log reductions due to additional treatments that increased product purity. A log reduction of nearly 7 orders of magnitude by sterilization of medical devices was estimated by the expert group likely due to the heat treatment during standard autoclaving which would denature RNA viruses.

Even though leukoreduction is already in place in Canada, which would significantly reduce XMRV, the deferral of CFS patients was implemented as a precautionary measure. A similar measure was implemented in some other countries (for example, Australia and the United Kingdom).[6]

8. Disease relationships (causal and non-causal)

The probability of XMRV and its causal linkage to prostate cancer resulted in a lack of consensus from the expert group. The heterogeneity of prostate cancers was not considered. While XMRV nucleic acid and protein had not been isolated from the blood of prostate cancer patients it was found in about 1% of stromal cells, predominantly fibroblasts and hematopoietic elements in regions adjacent to the carcinoma (Urisman et al., 2006). Similarly, the experts indicated a low probability of association between XMRV and CFS but this was also associated with significant uncertainty.   At the time of the meeting with high uncertainty surrounding XMRV as a potential emerging pathogen, the experts were very careful when interpreting and extrapolating the available research data. They acknowledged that the identification of XMRV RNA sequences in patient specimens by PCR assays was reported in the literature but it did not establish that infections had occurred and it did not prove disease causation or association with specific diseases. At this meeting some experts speculated about the possibility of sample contamination suggesting it may have occurred leading to contradictory cohort data. One important question that the experts agreed required more research was whether XMRV infection was a causal factor in the etiology of some CFS and prostate cancer cases or whether XMRV was merely a "passenger virus" identified in some healthy individuals and a subset of immunocompromised patient groups (e.g., CFS patients). Overall, the experts agreed that given the current understanding of XMRV that there was a very low probability that XMRV was implicated in disease etiology.

---

[6] For the Australian Red Cross Blood Service CFS deferral notice, see:

http://www.donateblood.com.au/media-centre/latest-national-news/blood-service-updates-cfs-donor-policy; for the United Kingdom National Health Service deferral notice see:

http://www.nhsbt.nhs.uk/news/2010/newsrelease071010.html.

9. Conclusions

The Krever Commission report (1997) acknowledged the benefits of using a reputable scientific evidence base when establishing public health policy to address any new emerging blood-borne pathogen in Canada. Krever concluded that, for emerging threats where there has been insufficient time to develop an adequate amount of scientific data to guide policy creation, such as those which periodically affect the blood supply, it is important to make the best possible effort to support policy making by means of qualitative and quantitative risk assessments in a timely manner (Krever, 1997; Wilson, 2007). Authorities should act even if there is only a theoretical risk of harm; and given the potential risk of an emerging pathogen regulators must err on the side of caution. Early on, in the absence of clear evidence, a precautionary approach for blood and CTO safety should be applied. Thus, the overarching guiding policy for any emerging pathogen should be the use of a precautionary approach.

As a result, Canadian regulators have adopted precautionary approaches in response to emerging and low probability but high consequence risk issues. The emergence of XMRV as a potential pathogen transmissible by blood resulted in a proactive and rapid response by Canadian risk managers and blood providers. In Canada a precautionary CFS blood deferral policy was put in place a few months prior to the expert meeting but at the time of the expert meeting the situation for CTO transplants remained an issue with uncertainty.

Risk management of emerging infectious retroviruses, such as XMRV, requires obtaining the needed contextual information, evidence (prevalence and incidence rates) and analyzing risk factors. Resources drawn upon include consultation with domestic experts, reviewing published and grey literature, awareness of global experience including accessing international expert opinion, utilizing available surveillance data, developing risk modeling with available data and considering other population health considerations.

During the 2009-2010 time period when high uncertainty existed surrounding XMRV the meeting helped to quantify knowledge gaps through the use of expert opinion. There was no direct evidence to support XMRV transmission through blood or CTOs; however, its detection in plasma and PBMCs of individuals in some studies suggested that these routes of transmission may be possible, and could significantly increase the risk to CTO recipients of exposure to this virus. The risks posed by XMRV to blood recipients would depend on its ability to cause diseases in humans, and the magnitude of this risk depends on whether only a subset of recipients (e.g., immunocompromised individuals) are susceptible to XMRV infection and disease or not. The route of transmission for any emerging blood-borne pathogen is dependent on the characteristics of the virus and the tissues affected.

The general population could potentially be exposed to a new emerging pathogen such as XMRV by various modes including vertical or horizontal transmission, as well as transmission through transfusion and transplantation. The detection of XMRV in plasma and PBMCs of infected individuals (Lombardi et al., 2009; Lo et al., 2010) suggested that there may be the possibility of a blood-borne transmission during transfusion. It was of concern that XMRV as an emerging pathogen might be transmitted through other body fluids such as semen and breast milk although there was no direct evidence to support these as routes of infection. The expert pairwise comparison exercise confirmed that there was good agreement that these other routes were a low risk probability for XMRV transmission.

Regulation for CTOs used for transplantation in Canada, came into effect in early 1999. The regulations minimize the potential health risks to Canadian recipients of human CTOs by providing safety and processing requirements including: donor screening, donor testing, sample collection and retrieval, preservation, packaging, labelling, and quarantine), storage, record keeping, distribution, importation, error, accident and adverse reaction investigation and reporting.

At the time of the expert meeting the lack of scientific consensus regarding the association of XMRV with CFS in available published studies complicated the response for many countries and often polarized the experts from reaching consensus on XMRV issues under discussion at our meeting. Initially, contradictory reports were believed to be due to variation in the diagnosis of CFS patients, methodological variability between reported studies (use of PCR versus immunochemistry) and the use of differing and non-standardized samples or reagents. Later the contradictory reports were largely explained due to sample, tissue cell line and diagnostic kit contamination by mouse nucleic acids or VP62 plasmid.

Convening an expert group and soliciting the best available unbiased advice on uncertainty gaps provides a measure of due diligence and attentiveness to virtual surveillance for an emerging CTO and blood risk. Experts indicated that for any emerging pathogen further studies would be needed to address the gaps in information in order to appropriately assess the risk of transfusion transmitted infections. Generically, this would require three main activities: First, the development of standardized, well validated tests and methods to determine the prevalence of the pathogen in the general population and in blood donors. Secondly, research investigating its mode of transmission and different routes of transmission are important to initiate; and thirdly, further research and evidence confirming the pathogen's role in human disease (if it is not already established) is required.

As a case study XMRV exemplified an emerging potential blood-borne pathogen and how Canadian decision-makers implemented a precautionary approach. At the time there was significant uncertainty over the identified knowledge gaps discussed by the experts. At the time of the meeting the experts suggested that establishing the prevalence in the adult general population and in at risk groups within a Canadian context were key experiments to consider. This applies to XMRV or other emerging pathogens that may affect blood supplies.

We know now that the initial linkage of XMRV to CFS may have been due to sample contamination and false positives. At the time of these discussions the experts correctly believed that the uncertainty over XMRV would be resolved within the next two years from ongoing international research and publication of peer reviewed data. Virtual surveillance along with ongoing international expert consultation is necessary and vitally important to keep up-to-date about emerging blood-borne pathogens.

Finally, we note that the experts and decision-makers dealing with XMRV as an emerging threat to blood safety employed precautionary actions very early on. According to the Krever report every effort should be made to protect the blood supply, cells, tissues and organs from emerging blood-borne pathogens even if the risk remains largely unknown or a causal association with a disease state has not been established (Krever, 1997). XMRV turned out to be a contaminant; however, convening Canadian and international experts to discuss issues surrounding XMRV risk showed that, in Canada, when faced with uncertainty the use of precaution and mobilization of experts as discussed by Krever (1997) was put into full effect. These early interventions allowed for proactive management of this potential emerging blood borne threat.

10. Acknowledgements

This work was supported by the Public Health Agency of Canada and Health Canada. The following individuals participated in the expert discussions on XMRV: Steve Anderson, Michael P. Busch, Rika A. Furuta, Jerry Holmberg, Éric Jeziorski, Harvey Klein, Judy Mikovits, Robert Silverman, Jonathan Stoye, Cees L. Van der Poel, Margaret Fearon, Marc Germain, Paul Jolicoeur, Bruce Ritchie, and Anton Andonov. We also thank: Tom Wong, Anil Dudani, Suja Mani, and Caroline Desjardins from the Public Health Agency of Canada for their ongoing support of this work.

11. References

Andonov A. 2010. "Screening for X/P-MLV Related Virus Sequences in Healthy Controls and Patients with Multiple Blood Transfusions". Public Health Agency of Canada, National Microbiology Laboratory, Ottawa, Canada. September 27, personal communication.

Aspinall W. 2010. A route to more tractable expert advice. Nature. 463(7279):294-5.

Bacich DJ, Sobek KM, Cummings JL, Atwood AA, and O'Keefe DS. 2011. False negative results from using common PCR reagents. BMC Res Notes. 4(1):457.

Carlowe J. 2010. Chronic fatigue syndrome is not caused by XMRV virus, study shows. BMJ. 341:c7358.

Carruthers BM, Jain AK, De Meirleir KL, Peterson DL, Klimas NG, Lerner AM, Bested AC, Flor-Henry P, Joshi P, Powles ACP, Sherkey JA, and van de Sande MI. 2003. Myalgic encephalomyelitis/chronic fatigue syndrome: clinical working case definition, diagnostic and treatment protocols. Journal of Chronic Fatigue Syndrome. 11:7–116.

Cohen J. 2011. More Negative Data for Link Between Mouse Virus and Human Disease. 331: 1253-54.

Fukuda K, Straus SE, Hickie I, Sharpe MC, Dobbins JG, and Komaroff AL. 1994. The chronic fatigue syndrome: a comprehensive approach to its definition and study. Ann Intern Med. 121:953-9.

Groom HC, Boucherit VC, Makinson K, Randal E, Baptista S, Hagan S, Gow JW, Mattes FM, Breuer J, Kerr JR, Stoye JP, and Bishop KN. 2010. Absence of xenotropic murine leukemia virus-related virus in UK patients with chronic fatigue syndrome. Retrovirology. 7:10.

Health Canada. 1998. Directive D98-01: Implementation of Prestorage Leukoreduction of Cellular Blood Components, Nov. 2, 1998. Available at: http://www.hc-sc.gc.ca/dhp-mps/alt_formats/hpfb-dgpsa/pdf/brgtherap/leukoreduction-deleucocytation-eng.pdf.

Holmes GP, Kaplan JE, Gantz NM, Komaroff AL, Schonberger LB, Straus SE, Jones JF, Dobois RE, Cunningham-Rundles C, Pahwa S, Tosato G, Zegans LS, Purtilo DT, Brown N, Schooley RT, and Brus I. 1988. Chronic fatigue syndrome: a working case definition. Ann Intern Med. 108:387-9.

Hong P, Li J, and Li Y. 2010. Failure to detect xenotropic murine leukemia virus-related virus in Chinese patients with chronic fatigue syndrome. Virol J. 7:224.

Hue S, Gray ER, Gall A, Katzourakis A, Tan CP, Houldcroft CJ, McLaren S, Pillay D, Futreal A, Garson JA, Pybus OG, Kellam P, and Towers GJ. 2010. Disease-associated XMRV sequences are consistent with laboratory contamination. Retrovirology. 7:111.

Kaiser J. 2011. Chronic fatigue syndrome. Studies point to possible contamination in XMRV findings. Science. 331(6013):17.

Knox K, Carrigan D, Simmons G, Teque F, Zhou Y, Hackett J Jr, Qiu X, Luk KC, Schochetman G, Knox A, Kogelnik AM, and Levy JA. 2011. No evidence of murine-like gammaretroviruses in CFS patients previously identified as XMRV-infected. Science. 333(6038):94-7.

Krever H. 1997. Volume 3: Chapter 40, The Blood System of the Future. Commission of Inquiry on the Blood System in Canada, Krever Commission. Canada, Public Works and Government Services Canada, Ottawa, Ontario.

Lo S-C, Pripuzova N, Bingjie L, Komaroff AL, Hung G-C, Wang R, and Alter H. 2010. Detection of MLV-related gag gene sequences in blood of patients with chronic fatigue syndrome and healthy blood donors. Proc Natl Acad Sci U S A. 107:15874-9.

Lombardi VC, Ruscetti FW, Das Gupta J, Pfost MA, Hagen KS, Peterson DL, Ruscetti SK, Bagni RK, Petrow-Sadowski C, Gold B, Dean M, Silverman RH, and Mikovits JA. 2009. Detection of an infectious retrovirus, XMRV, in blood cells of patients with chronic fatigue syndrome. Science. 326:585-9.

Macutkiewicz M. 2008. Paired comparisons and group preference. Master of Science Thesis, Unpublished. Applied Mathematics Risk and Environmental Modeling, TU Delft; 92pp.

Oakes B, Tai AK, Cingoz O, Henefield MH, Levine S, Coffin JM, and Huber BT. 2010. Contamination of human DNA samples with mouse DNA can lead to false detection of XMRV-like sequences. Retrovirology. 7:109.

Paprotka T, Delviks-Frankenberry KA, Cingöz O, Martinez A, Kung HJ, Tepper CG, Hu WS, Fivash MJ Jr, Coffin JM, and Pathak VK. 2011. Recombinant origin of the retrovirus XMRV. Science. 333(6038):97-101.

Xenotropic Murine Leukemia Virus-Related Virus as a Case Study: Using a Precautionary Risk Management
Approach for Emerging Blood-Borne Pathogens in Canada

107

Reeves WC, Wagner D, Nisenbaum R, Jones JF, Gurbaxani B, Solomon L, Papanicolaou DA, Unger ER, Vernon SD, and Heim C. 2005. Chronic fatigue syndrome-a clinically empirical approach to its definition and study. BMC Med. 3:19.

Robinson MJ, Erlwein OW, Kaye S, Weber J, Cingoz O, Patel A,Walker MM, Kim W-J, Uiprasertkul M, Coffin JM and McClure MO. 2010. Mouse DNA contamination in human tissue tested for XMRV. Retrovirology. 7:108.

Sato E, Furuta RA, and Miyazawa T. 2010. An endogenous murine leukemia viral genome contaminant in a commercial RTPCR Kit is amplified using standard primers for XMRV. Retrovirology. 7:110.

Schlaberg R, Choe DJ, Brown KR, Thaker HM, and Singh IR. 2009. XMRV is present in malignant prostatic epithelium and is associated with prostate cancer, especially high-grade tumors. Proceedings of the National Academy of Sciences, U S A. 106:16351-16356.

Sharpe MC, Archard LC, Banatvala JE, Borysiewica LK, Clare AW, David A, Edwards RH, Hawton KE, Lambert HP, and Lane RJ. 1991. A report - chronic fatigue syndrome: guidelines for research. J Royal Soc Med. 84:118-21.

Silverman RH, Das Gupta J, Lombardi VC, Ruscetti FW, Pfost MA, Hagen KS, Peterson DL, Ruscetti SK, Bagni RK, Petrow-Sadowski C, Gold B, Dean M, Mikovits JA. 2011. Partial retraction. Detection of an infectious retrovirus, XMRV, in blood cells of patients with chronic fatigue syndrome. Science. 334(6053):176.

Smith RA. 2010. Contamination of clinical specimens with MLV-encoding nucleic acids: implications for XMRV and other candidate human retroviruses. Retrovirology. 7:112.

Switzer WM, Jia H, Hohn O, Zheng H, Tang S, Shankar A, Bannert N, Simmons G, Hendry RM, Falkenberg VR, Reeves WC, and Heneine W. 2010. Absence of evidence of xenotropic murine leukemia virus-related virus infection in persons with chronic fatigue syndrome and healthy controls in the United States. Retrovirology. 7:57.

Tuke PW, Tettmar KI, Tamuri A, Stoye JP, and Tedder RS. 2011. PCR master mixes harbour murine DNA sequences. Caveat emptor! PLoS One. 6(5):e19953.

Tyshenko MG, ElSaadany S, Oraby T, Darshan S, Aspinall W, Cooke R, Catford A and Krewski D. 2011. Expert Elicitation for the Judgment of Prion Disease Risk Uncertainties, Journal of Toxicology and Environmental Health, Part A. 74(2): 261-285.

Urisman A, Molinaro RJ, Fischer N, Plummer SJ, Casey G, Klein EA, Malathi K, Magi-Galluzzi C, Tubbs RR, Ganem D, Silverman RH, and DeRisi JL. 2006. Identification of a novel gammaretrovirus in prostate tumors of patients homozygous for R462Q RNASEL variant. PLoS Pathogen. 2(3):e25.

van Kuppeveld FJ, de Jong AS, Lanke KH, Verhaegh GW, Melchers WJ, Swanink CM, Bleijenberg G, Netea MG, Galama JM, and van der Meer JW. 2010. Prevalence of xenotropic murine leukemia virus-related virus in patients with chronic fatigue syndrome in the Netherlands: retrospective analysis of samples from an established cohort. Br Med J. 340.

Wilson K, Wilson M, Hébert PC, and Graham I. 2003. The application of the precautionary principle to the blood system: the Canadian blood system's vCJD donor deferral policy. Transfus Med Rev. 17(2): 89-94.

Wilson K. 2007. The Krever Commission-10 years later. CMAJ. 177: 1387-1389.

Yang J, Battacharya P, Singhal R, and Kandel1 ES. 2011. Xenotropic murine leukemia virus-related virus (XMRV) in prostate cancer cells likely represents a laboratory artifact Oncotarget 2011. 2: 358-362.

Part 3

Improving Future Risk Assessment Analyses

6

Physics of Open Systems: A New Approach to Use Genomics Data in Risk Assessment

Viacheslav Ageev[1], Boric Fomin[1], Oleg Fomin[1], Tamara Kachanova[1],
Chao Chen[2], Maria Spassova[2] and Leonid Kopylev[2]
[1]Faculty of Innovations, Saint-Petersburg State Polytechnic University
[2]National Center for Environmental Assessment, Office of Research and Development
Environmental Protection Agency
[1]Russia
[2]USA

1. Introduction

Modern genomics technologies allow acquisition of huge volumes of gene expression data of the whole genome of different biological systems. It has created a new platform for understanding the exposure effects of toxic stressors on biological systems, for discovering the genetic markers of the negative impact of toxicants, for identifying the potential hazards, and for increasing the precision and efficiency of risk assessment.

Biological processes preceding the appearance of observable harmful effects due to exposures to a toxic chemical are very complex. Recognizing these biological processes as an early response is a key element in increasing the sensitivity of hazard and dose-response assessments for environmental agents. Such processes might be detectable at lower doses and may help to identify a hazard at a low-dose region that is relevant to environmental exposures. An important but often controversial issue in risk assessment is the shape of the dose-response curve at low doses: for example, is there a threshold effect? In the absence of sufficient scientific information, linear and non-threshold effects are assumed as the default position in the U.S. Environmental Protection Agency (EPA) cancer risk assessments (US EPA, 2005). Most attempts to establish a threshold effect were based on traditional toxicological data from animal bioassays, and *in vivo* and *in vitro* experiments for mode of action (MOA) studies that may involve animal or human cell cultures. Formaldehyde provides a good example to show how attempts have been made to evaluate effects at low doses (Conolly et al., 2004) and how uncertain they can be (Crump et al., 2008).

Emerging data from toxicogenomic studies has raised hope that the data may provide useful information about the shape of dose-response at low doses. Bioinformatics methods that can be used for dose-response analysis of high dimensional, multiple factors data are quite limited but are critically needed. Yu et al. (2006) introduced a method to apply Gene Ontology (GO) analysis to dose-response studies. Thomas et al. (2007) applied benchmark dose (BMD) tools (Crump, 1984) and BMD software (US EPA, 2006) to analyze such data. Using micro-array expression data from rats exposed to formaldehyde by inhalation for 6 hours at 0, 0.7, 2.0, 6.0, and 15 ppm, Thomas et al. (2007) identified a subset of genes that shows a non-linear dose-response relationship with a non-significant gene activity at and below 6 ppm, implying a potential threshold effect. This dose-response behavior is similar to that of rat nasal tumors from inhaled formaldehyde which showed a very steep dose response (Kerns et al., 1983; Monticello et al., 1996). The subset of genes identified in Thomas et al. (2007) is obtained by test of statistically significant difference from the control using one-way analysis of variance. The identified subset of genes may be responsible for the observed tumors at high doses. However, it is possible that there is another subset of genes that may represent the MOA at low doses. Thus, the controversy about the shape of dose-response at low doses remains unless a unique MOA can be established for both low and high doses.

The Physics of Open Systems (PS) is an approach (Kachanova & Fomin, 2010) that is able to reveal the complexity of a bio-system. This paper introduces methods and technologies of PS and provides examples of its use in generation of system knowledge about gene expression on the basis of genomics microarray data. Methods of PS are applied to studying effects of bio-systems chemical exposure by analysis of genomic data. A detailed analysis of the Thomas et al. (2007) data using the PS approach is presented. The results are compared to the results from the original study and some advantages of the PS method are revealed.

2. Physics of open systems

Ideas and methods of PS are realized in the information technologies by providing complexity reduction and reconstruction of the whole empirical information in an open system (Kachanova & Fomin, 1999, 2002, 2003, 2009). Systemological concepts of PS were formed by solving a general problem of reconstructive analysis of complex systems by their empirical descriptions; this solution led to creation of a new method of obtaining scientific knowledge on open systems (*http://isd-consortium.ru/*). Theoretical basis of PS was formed as a result of creating a language of open system and qualimetry (measuring quality) of system knowledge. Development of the language of systems leads to understanding and rational explanation of obtained knowledge. PS is considered completed after the solution to the problem of synthesis of open systems is discovered. Based on this solution, the method is created for modeling states and for discovering emergent (means properties belonging only to the system; could not be derived of individual parts of a system in final number of steps) properties and patterns of an open system.

The PS-based solution for systems research applied problems is accomplished through performing the highly automated technological cycle including five subcomponents: (1) PS technology of context formation transforms experimental data into a format that is used in PS for initial empirical description of the systems; (2) PS technology of system reconstructions builds, based on empirical description of the system, its abstract representation by signed connection graph. The connection graph reflects characteristic for open systems heterogeneity of structures, states, and behavior of the system. This technology generates, based on connection graph, a family of formal system models that reveals the complexity of open systems in a family of its unique qualities. A family of such models contains system knowledge on structural invariants, behavioral invariants, roles and activities of parameters; (3) PS technology of system examination assesses sufficiency of empirical description for construction of complete set of system models, determines degree of completeness of each system model, constructs and verifies invariants of ideal system states; (4) PS technology of system design generates reconstructions of actual system states. System reconstructions serve as base for obtaining knowledge on system mechanisms that explain magnitude and characteristic changes of parameters in each system state; and (5) PS technology of pattern formation transforms system knowledge into solutions of applied problems (Kachanova & Fomin, 1999).

2.1 Technology of context formation

PS technology of context formation represents the system in data obtained by observing and measuring interactions of the system with the environment. The system, in its natural scale and complexity, maps onto empirical description (empirical context). PS works best with complete empirical contexts. The key object of this technology is the empirical context of the system in the format of tabulated observations. In genomics, each row of the table describes states of one bio-object at given experimental conditions. Each column of the table contains particular gene levels of expression. The table size can be in tens, hundreds or thousands. The result of the technology is representation of a system in a space of its attributes. The coordinates of this space are represented by genes, and points of the space are states of bio-system.

2.2 Technology of system reconstructions

PS technology of system reconstruction automatically produces system knowledge based on empirical description of the system (Kachanova & Fomin, 2003). The empirical description is then transformed into abstract representation of the system in a form of signed connections graph (Fig. 1). The graph vertices are genes. The graph connections are statistically significant binary relationships ($p<0.05$). The edges have several attributes: strength, sign, and monotonicity (homotypic character of changes in gene expressions). These attributes are computed based on several different statistical approaches: Shannon index (Shannon, 1948), Kendall rank correlation coefficient (Kendall, 1970), Hoeffding independence test, and Blum-Kiefer-Rosenblatt independence test (Hollander & Wolfe, 1999). The structure of the binary relationships represents multiplicity of intra-system correlations. The signs of the binary relationships define different forms of system behavior.

The first axiom of PS (Kachanova & Fomin, 1999) states that changes in all system parameters are harmonic. The connection graph as representation of the system obtained from independently determined binary connections satisfies this axiom if all its cycles are even (signed balance). An out-of-balance condition of the connection graph shows heterogeneity of the system and its complexity. Connection graph with signs out-of-balance serves as a base for an automatic generation of complete set of system models. Each model determines system in its one quality. A complete set of models determines all qualities of the system.

Generation of system models starts with the finding in connection graphs of all unbalanced triangles (Fig. 2). Each unbalanced triangle is a minimal structure of binary relationship of parameters with out-of-balance connections signs. A system needs to be discovered in all its qualities and each quality of the system has to be homogeneous. Resolving lack of balance in the connection graph is realized in PS by finding symmetries of structures of relationships – singletons with the ability to harmonize connections between parameters (Kachanova & Fomin, 1999). A singleton is an unbalanced triangle with axial symmetry and system roles of vertices. One vertex is special and identifies a quality of the system. Two other vertices serve as system-forming two-factor interaction. Vertices that belong to at least one singleton have leading system role. All singletons with the same special vertex form a kernel of system model with preservation of axial symmetry and two-factor relationships. The kernel determines a single quality of the system. System model with such a kernel represents the system as a whole in its one quality. The system as a whole in all its qualities is represented by the complete set of system models (Fig. 2). This complete set discovers complexity of the system.

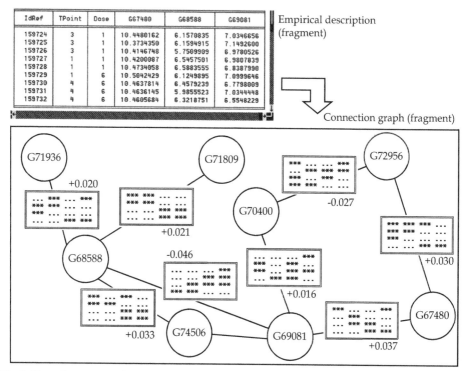

Fig. 1. Transformation of the empirical context into connection graph. Graph vertices are probes. Graph connections are statistically significant binary relationships with attributes: strength, sign, and monotonicity.

The result of PS technology is knowledge on space of qualities of the system which are images of family of abstract system models. Each system model matches a region in which particular quality of the system is represented. The structure of the region determines conceptual borders showing qualities with different intensity.

2.3 Technology of system examination

PS technology of system examination assesses generated system knowledge and constructs, based on system models, a complete set of ideal states of the system. It also maps each region of the space of qualities into the space of attributes and determines set of objects with

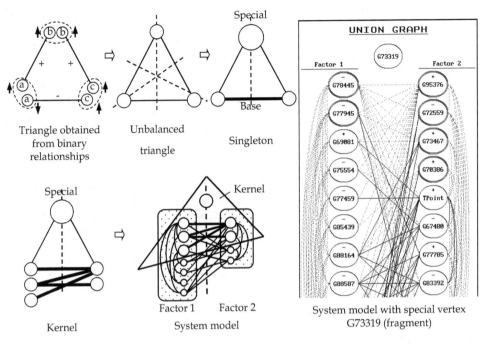

Fig. 2. Schematic description of a system model: finding in connection graphs all unbalanced triangles; determining singletons; obtaining kernel of a system model; building up factors of the system model by inclusion of vertices from the kernel neighborhood; and forming a system model.

quality characteristics for this region. The technology works with words, concepts and assessments of the language of systems (Kachanova & Fomin, 2009). It uses these objects to represent properties of each system using generated system knowledge.

The technology works with different forms of representation of the system: empirical description; complete set of system models; system model of each quality; and complete family of condensed triangles (condensed is in the same sense as condensed graph). For each system representation there is a special approach of assessing the properties of that representation. The technology obtains assessments of system properties of parameters, the structure of binary relationships, and system models. With this as a base, the technology constructs complex assessments of complex properties of the system. For comparative analysis, the technology introduces and uses preference relations and the rule of group choices.

The empirical description of the system is assessed based on its sufficiency for generation of complete system knowledge. In the complete system knowledge, heterogeneity of the system is completely revealed: unbalances are resolved, and changes in all parameters are explained by system mechanisms. The family of system models is assessed by its ability to express completely the space of system qualities. Each system model is characterized by absolute assessments of its ability to represent characteristic quality of the system. To determine these assessments, the technology constructs a basic sample of the system model (the ideal representation of sense of qualitative determinacy in an abstract form). For this sample, assessments of shapeness and homogeneity are computed. The shapeness is determined by the morphological characteristics of the sample. The homogeneity characterizes conceptual equivalency of all parts of the basic sample. The condensed triangle is the ultimate concentrated image of a system quality expressed by a system model. The condensed triangle serves as an instrument that maps a region of the space of qualities into the space of attributes of the system. For assessment of the quality of the condensed triangle, the technology introduces complex quantitative characteristics of adequacy of representation of a system model in the condensed triangle.

The main purpose of technology of system examination is transformation of the family of system models into a set of models of the ideal states of the system. Main axial symmetry of a system model allows only two ways of concordance of its signs in agreement with the first axiom of PS. Each alternative gives rise to a model of stereotype of the system. The model of each stereotype is transformed into two models of ideal states of the system in accordance with the individualization axiom. This axiom establishes existence of a unique border between high and low values (Kachanova & Fomin, 1999). In a model of ideal state, each parameter obtains a level of value on a nominal scale High/Low. Two models of the ideal states of the same stereotype have the same signs of connections and opposite levels of the vertices values. Complete set of models of the ideal states determines the system as a whole with all its qualities and all ways of manifestation of these qualities in reality.

The direct mapping of regions of the space of system qualities into its space of attributes is achieved by mapping of the set of models of the ideal states on the empirical description of the system. This mapping is achieved by using condensed triangles and special scales of numerical levels of parameters values. The technology constructs scale for each parameter in each ideal model. Each parameter that possesses nominal level (High/Low) obtains a quantitative level. The set of all quantitative levels of parameters determines region of the ideal in the space of attributes. This region contains set of objects whose states correspond to that ideal with different intensity of manifestation of qualities of the ideal in reality. A set of such objects forms cluster of experimental objects (Fig. 3).

Joint set of singletons, system models, and models of the ideal states form complete layout of the system in which concepts of the system are given and revealed in abstract representations. The result of the technology of system examination is knowledge on the quality of the empirical description, the quality of all system and ideal models, and the quality of maps of regions of the qualities space into the space of attributes. The empirical description quality conceptualizes and assesses the system from the position of changing values and features of their correlations. The quality of the model assesses its shapeness, homogeneity, completeness, and ability to completely reveal and correctly transfer concepts of the system to observed data. The quality of mapping provides ability of forming sets of clusters to represent all system concepts revealed in each model of the ideal state.

2.4 Technology of system design

PS technology of system design applies set of clusters for construction of models of observed states. Each ideal state of the system is realized in different experimental objects with different intensity. On the basis of each set of clusters, the technology generates models

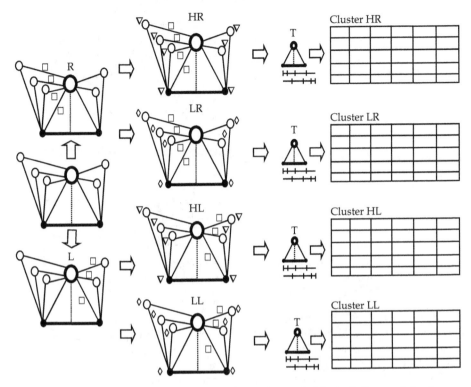

Fig. 3. Schematic of construction of clusters of experimental objects: R, L – models of stereotypes of system behavior; HR, LR, HL, LL – models of ideal states; «□» – balanced model; «∇» – balanced model with special vertex at High level; «◊» – balanced model with special vertex at Low level; and «T» – condensed triangle with numerical levels of values. Cluster is the set of experimental objects corresponding to the model of the ideal state of the system.

of implementation forms of the ideal. Such model includes cluster of experimental objects and assessments of degree of implementation of the ideal in these objects. Objects in the cluster occupy certain region in the space of system attributes generated by the ideal model. The ideal also belongs to this region. The degree of 'closeness' of each object in the cluster to the ideal is determined by a special 'closeness' scale. The ability of each parameter of the state associated with experimental objects to transfer systemic concept of the ideal is assessed by a set of values on quantitative scales (Fig. 4).

The main purpose of the technology of system design is automatic generation of reconstructions of actual system states that are represented in the system empirical description by states of experimental objects. The model of implementation forms of each ideal contains a cluster with experimental objects associated with that ideal. The result of the direct mapping of the ideal onto empirical description of the system is a set of clusters of objects which have intersections. All objects from the empirical description represent states of the system. All objects from each cluster represent different states from the position of one system quality.

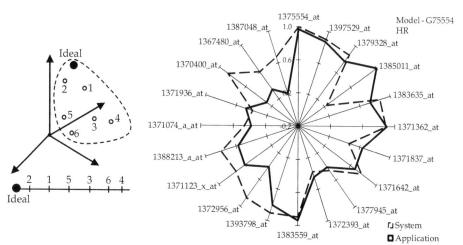

Fig. 4. Attributes of model of implementation forms of the ideal: measure of 'closeness' to ideal on scale of 'closeness' and system significance and application significance of parameters of the ideal model.

Each observed state of the system corresponds to a particular set of models of the implementation forms of different ideals. The reconstruction of implemented state appears as a result of assembly of all models of the given set. In a model of the ideal state, the system has one quality, generated by two-factor interaction that forms the kernel of the system model from singleton with common axial symmetry. In the reconstruction of the implemented state the system is (as a result of that assembly) multi-quality and generated by interactions that form the kernel of the model of the reconstruction from singletons of the ideal models. The kernel of the model reconstruction has not only axial symmetry of singletons but also all symmetries of the higher order, which harmonize qualities that form particular state of the system (Fig. 5).

The states of the system are revealed in reconstructions by parameters and mechanisms that characterize and determine these states. Each parameter has a set of attributes that are assessed from the position of the system as a whole by special quantitative scales. In an observed state of the system, each parameter of the state has a certain value on the measuring scale. In models of the ideal states all parameters are determined on levels High or Low. In models of implementation forms of the ideal states, the levels of parameters are assigned to levels High or Low with a degree of revealing intensity for this level. In the reconstruction of states of the observation, each parameter can be differently determined by different models of implementation forms (some model forms assess value as Low with some intensity and some as High with some intensity). Resolving such uncertainty is achieved by the scale of level prevalence. Each parameter of the state obtains a level on the ordinal 17-item scale. Each item of the scale matches certain intensity of manifestation of high, medium, low values of the parameter. In PS, special numeric scales are constructed based on Farey sums (Conway & Guy, 1996) and Saaty (1980) scale. The stability of parameter level in each observed state is assigned a value on the ordinal 4-item scale – the scale of predeterminacy.

System model	Objects (2 ppm, 6 hours)			
	GSM159757	GSM159758	GSM159759	GSM159760
G77945	HR	LL	LL	LL
G95990	HR	HR	HL	HL
G85439	HR		HR	LL
G74517	HL		LR	HR
G78445	HL		LR	LR
G79201	HL	HL		LL
G87048	HL	LR	LR	
G76337		LR	HR	LR
G75599	HR			HL
G97551	HR			LR
G97697	HR			HL
G73097	HR			LR

Fig. 5. Reconstructions of states (fragment): The tabular representation of models of reconstructions of four objects; cells of the table show codes of ideal states of system models; and drawing of kernel of model reconstruction of one object.

The mechanism that forms observed state of the system appears as a result of assembly of mechanisms represented by a set of models of implementation forms of the ideals. In the reconstruction of the observed state, each particular system mechanism assists in confirmation or changes of this state. The role of each mechanism in determination of this state is done by the reconstruction of the observed state. For mechanisms with role in changes of the state, it is determined along which parameters and directions these changes do happen. The complete set of reconstructions contains knowledge of all system as a whole and its emergent properties. Thus it represents knowledge on limitations and patterns of conjugacy on different qualities of the system in their observed states. The results of the technology are models of rational explanation of properties of each parameter in each state; properties of system as a whole; properties of observed states of the system as a whole; and mechanisms that form changes of each parameter and of global system properties.

2.5 Technology of pattern formation

PS technology of pattern formation works with the obtained system knowledge. It transforms system knowledge into informational, intellectual, cognitive, and technological resources of knowledge that serve as instruments of solving typical applied problems. Informational resource is knowledge that is the product of the system analysis and conceptualization of empirical facts (deficiencies and assessments of the quality of the empirical description, level of importance of the parameters, and relevancy of the parameters and the experimental objects to the problems that need solutions). The intellectual resource consists of the family of formal models that generate cognitive potential for research (system models as well as assessments of completeness of the system knowledge). The cognitive resource is the knowledge that serves for reasoning and action that has translational potential and provides generation of universally-notional ways of scientific communication such as models, objects, schematics, and language of systems. The technological resource is the objective knowledge on the system as a whole and its parts that allows rational explanation of system states and mechanisms of system changes (states and the space of states). The technology of pattern formation actualizes, organizes, and offers formed knowledge resources for the solution of applied systemic problems.

The technology of pattern formation transforms resources of knowledge into formats that could be applied for solution of applied problems. When working with genomic data, technology accounts for features of empirical descriptions of bio-systems: missing data, data on replicated experiments, and possibly insufficient representativeness. To establish patterns, formats are used in such a way that elements of the knowledge are represented in the special scales allowing for recovery of missing data, aggregation of levels, generalization of levels, and 3-item scale. In reconstructions of the states, levels of the parameters are determined by the system mechanisms. This allows creation of scale that allows recovering levels of values of missing data. Reconstruction of states models observed values of parameters by levels of their values on 17-items scale of level prevalence. Set of levels of the parameters obtained in replicated experiments is represented by an item on 13-item scale of level aggregation. This scale is effective for homogeneous data, because levels from the set lie in one zone of the scale of level prevalence. When data is not homogeneous, aggregation may be achieved by application of the scale of generalized levels. If heterogeneity is prominent, this scale results in level uncertainty. 3-item scale is a simplification of these scales. On 3-item scale, each region of high, medium, and low values obtains item of the scale (H, M, L).

The technology of pattern formation uses, in application to the type of parameters changes caused by external influences, technological resource and, accounting for features of the empirical material, develops methods of solving problems based on the obtained knowledge.

3. Profiles of gene activity for rats exposed to formaldehyde

3.1 Empirical description of GO-categories

The experimental data on gene expressions of rats exposed to formaldehyde (http://www.ncbi.nlm.nih.gov/geo/query/acc.cgi?acc=GSE7002) are used in this article to illustrate how PS can be used to analyze this type of data. There were 90 rats total (including 25 in the control group). Parameters of the experiment are formaldehyde concentration exposure at various levels (0; 0.7; 2; 6; 15 ppm) and variable sacrifice times (6 hours; 24 hours; 5 days; 8 days; and 19 days) (See Table 1).

Formaldehyde concentration, ppm	Time					Total
	6 hours	24 hours	5 days	8 days	19 days	
0	8	4	4	5	4	25
0.7	4	4	4	4	4	20
2	4	4	5	4	4	21
6	4	4	4	4	4	20
15	4	-	-	-	-	4
Total	24	16	17	17	16	90

Table 1. Number of rats in each experimental group.

Thomas et al. (2007) conducted the experiment and analyzed the genomics data statistically. This article presents results of system analysis of the genomic data by PS methods.

Gene populations were structured according to NTNU GeneTools ontology (http://www.genetools.microarray.ntnu.no) that contains biological, molecular, and cellular components. GO-categories, containing certain sets of genes, correspond to hierarchical structure from each part of ontology. In each GO-category, genes are endowed by systemic homogeneity. This allows for the consideration of each GO-category as a system and thus allows investigation of rat gene expressions by PS methods. These methods are used to resolve changes in gene expressions for genes from four GO-categories (Table 2). The two GO-categories from the biological process ontology are traditionally thought to be related to formaldehyde MOA (e.g. Thomas et al., 2007). The empirical description of each GO-category as a system is a table with rows showing experimental bio-objects (rats), and column showing values of gene expressions.

Ontology	ID of GO-category	Name of GO-category	Level in hierarchy	Number of genes
Molecular function	GO:0004386	Helicase activity	3	118
Biological process	GO:0006281	DNA repair	6	204
	GO:0006954	Inflammatory response	5	281
Cellular component	GO:0016604	Nuclear body	6	119

Table 2. Description of GO-categories.

3.2 System models

The empirical description of GO-category serves as an initial representation of the system in data; the technology of system reconstructions transforms it into attributed connection graph. The connection graph reveals the complexity (heterogeneity) characteristic of the bio-systems (Table 3). Each significant binary connection in a connection graph serves as projection of multiple intra-system correlations. Heterogeneity of the system is transferred by the population of all binary connections which mostly are weak and complex, resulting in a large number of unbalanced triangles.

Based on the connection graph of the GO-category, the technology of system reconstructions obtains complete family of the system models that reveal system complexity of that GO-category. Each model of this family is generated by the same scheme. All GO-categories are complex systems (Table 4).

The characteristic of heterogeneity of systems is number of the system models and is comprised of number of singletons describing a GO-category. The complexity of each GO-category is completely revealed in the system models. This is confirmed by the high fraction of unbalanced triangles with resolved unbalance (carriers of heterogeneity of the system). The family of the system models determines changes in all parameters with leading system role. In the opposite case, the system knowledge on pattern of changes in the models is not completely revealed. Such a deficiency of the system knowledge may be caused by incomplete representativeness or possible incompleteness of empirical contexts.

3.3 Quality of system knowledge

The system knowledge is represented by families of system models. The technology of system examination provides assessment of the quality of system knowledge (Table 5).

GO-category	Total number of connections	Connection measures		Connection Sign		Connection Strength		Triangles	
		Informational	Nonparametric	Positive	Negative	Complex	Strong	Total	Unbalanced
GO:0004386	3307	1617	1690	2079	1225	1912	5	29368	4472
GO:0006281	9065	4312	4753	5559	3506	5251	0	135690	17730
GO:0006954	14990	7046	7944	10806	4184	8719	18	2858755	26132
GO:0016604	3282	1615	1667	1951	1327	1869	2	28983	3841

Table 3. Quantitative characteristics of connection graphs.

GO-category	Number of models	Number of singletons	Fraction of triangles with unbalance resolved	Leading system role of parameter, %
GO:0004386	126	1379	0.94	100
GO:0006281	209	3667	0.93	100
GO:0006954	275	4476	0.85	100
GO:0016604	123	1455	0.97	100

Table 4. Characteristics of system models.

GO-category	The ideal of expression of system concept		Expression of context in system models	
	Quality of shapeness	Quality of homogeneity	With good quality of shapeness, %	With good quality of homogeneity, %
GO:0004386	0.70	0.82	29	100
GO:0006281	0.58	0.78	56	100
GO:0006954	0.68	0.80	51	100
GO:0016604	0.64	0.79	73	100

Table 5. Integral assessments of quality of the system knowledge.

GO-category	Quality of condensed triangle	Direct mappings %	Volume of implemented concepts	Average number of ideals per object
GO:0004386	0.33	91	3159	35
GO:0006281	0.36	85	4143	46
GO:0006954	0.31	90	6606	73
GO:0016604	0.34	90	2945	33

Table 6. Integral assessments of qualities of direct mappings.

A fraction of models with good assessments is used as general characteristics of completeness and finality of the system knowledge. A system model completely responds to the ideal if assessments of shapeness and homogeneity equal to the scale value of 1. A model has a good quality if its scale value exceeds 0.6. The main problem of the technology of system examination is construction of the set of clusters of bio-objects that are carriers of a particular quality of the system (Table 6). The condensed triangle serves as a tool of direct mapping of the ideals of the system onto objects belonging to clusters. A condensed triangle is constructed for each ideal. Average assessment of quality of all condensed triangles is satisfactory (the mapping tool is adequate when assessment value is 0). Quality of direct mapping is satisfactory if more than 90% of the ideal states obtained empirical confirmation as adequate. The purpose of the direct mapping of the family of models of the ideal system states is determining the volume of system concepts, implemented in observed system states (total number of objects in all clusters is a summed number of system qualities that are associated with experimental animals). Volume of implemented concepts and the average number of the ideals per object reveals noticeable heterogeneity of mechanisms that form observed states of experimental animals (bio-objects).

3.4 Reconstructions of observed states

The technology of system design completes automatic generation of the system knowledge. It constructs models of observed states of bio-objects and assesses their quality (Table 7).

Reconstructions are constructed for all ninety experimental animals. The changes in all parameters for all observed states are determined by the revealed system mechanisms (values of all parameters-obtained explanation). For almost all parameters, the level of value can be established (with unique definition of levels of values on the scale of level prevalence). Pre-determinicity of levels of values by system mechanisms in all observed states is sufficiently high.

GO-category	Number of reconstructions	Determinicity, %	Supportability of the level, %	Pre-determinicity of the level
GO:0004386	90	98	97	84
GO:0006281	90	99	99.8	86
GO:0006954	90	98	98	85
GO:0016604	90	98	97	83

Table 7. Characteristics of states reconstructions.

For solving the problem of formaldehyde influence on changes in gene activity of bio-objects, reconstructions are used as the formal model that explains system patterns of joint harmonized changes of all parameters in each observed state. For each bio-object, each parameter obtains the level of value on the 17-item scale of level prevalence and value of the pre-determinicity attribute of that level (Table 8).

The observed values of each parameter in each observed state obtain formal definitions via sets of models of the system mechanisms that correspond to: determination of High and Low levels in a given state (class 1); formation of medium levels (class 2); determination of change potentials that explain type of changes in observed values (class 3). The quality of modeling experimental values of parameters by levels is estimated by the concordance coefficient (Fig. 6).

Factor	Value	Level	Pre-determinicity	Model classes		
				1	2	3
1375599_at	3.776569	15	High	G85779/LR	G75599/HR, G89389/LR	G74011/HL, G73256/HL
1397405_at	6.805443	4	High	G73557/LL		G71936/LR, G74342/HL, G97405/LR, G85276/HR, G88213/HR, G73256/HL
1371123_x_at	9.592442	10	Sufficient	G73557/LL, G85349/HR, G75554/HR	G85439/HR, G74332/LL, G72377/LL	G71936/LR, G74342/HL, G74011/HL, G75901/HL, G71123/HL, G88213/HR, G68619/HL
1371642_at	11.87329	9	High	G73557/LL, G85349/HR, G96713/HR, G75554/HR	G89389/LR, G72377/LL	G74342/HL, G77945/LL, G77459/HL, G75633/HL, G94383/HR, G71123/HL, G74470/LR, G88213/HR
1397551_at	7.676976	15	Sufficient	G73557/LL, G98472/HL, G81683/LR	G88864/LL, G97551/HR, G89389/LR, G74332/LL	G71936/LR, G75633/HL, G75901/HL, G73256/HL, G68619/HL
1370979_at	7.183854	7	Sufficient	G85349/HR, G98472/HL, G81683/LR	G72377/LL	G71936/LR, G77945/LL, G75901/HL, G71123/HL, G88213/HR, G68619/HL

Table 8. Reconstruction of observed states of bio-object GSM159785 (fragment). The last three columns: codes of models of system mechanisms (PS notation).

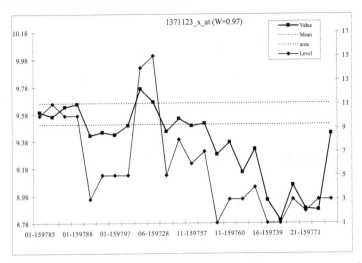

Fig. 6. Values of activity and levels of values for probe 1371123_x_at: x-axis – codes of objects; left y-axis – gene expression values; right y-axis – scale of level prevalence; and W – the concordance coefficient value.

Active probe set	Level of values	Formaldehyde concentration					Significance level	Transition type	Point of the first transition, ppm
		0 ppm 25 rats	0.7 ppm 20 rats	2 ppm 21 rats	6 ppm 20 rats	15 ppm 4 rats			
1367671_at	High	5	2	5	12	4	0.001	LH	6
	Low	9	8	8	1	0			
1368083_at	High	3	5	4	10	4	0.005	LH	6
	Low	10	7	8	2	0			
1368204_at	High	13	5	4	4	0	0.003	HL	2
	Low	1	4	10	8	2			
1368247_at	High	4	13	5	6	0	0.049	LHL	0.7
	Low	6	4	9	8	3			
1368311_at	High	11	9	4	6	0	0.021	HL	6
	Low	7	1	3	9	4			
1368410_at	High	8	8	6	4	0	0.016	HL	2
	Low	3	2	10	8	4			
1369965_at	High	13	8	4	2	0	0.000	HL	2
	Low	3	1	8	11	3			
1370910_at	High	10	9	5	3	0	0.042	HL	2
	Low	6	3	10	8	2			
1371217_at	High	2	9	6	3	4	0.036	C	0.7
	Low	6	4	7	8	0			
1371422_at	High	6	3	8	6	4	0.042	HLH	0.7
	Low	4	11	5	8	0			
1371911_at	High	4	4	8	8	4	0.021	LH	2
	Low	11	7	4	3	0			

1372181_at	High	8	8	5	4	0	0.028	HL	6
	Low	2	5	6	10	4			
1372393_at	High	7	7	6	3	4	0.040	HLH	6
	Low	6	3	9	10	0			
1372548_at	High	4	4	11	9	0	0.016	LHL	2
	Low	9	5	2	5	3			
1373094_at	High	3	5	6	10	4	0.048	LH	6
	Low	8	8	7	4	0			
1373280_at	High	8	5	4	6	4	0.021	HLH	2
	Low	2	3	11	8	0			
1373745_at	High	12	11	4	1	0	0.000	HL	2
	Low	4	1	8	10	3			
1374210_at	High	10	8	4	3	0	0.034	HL	2
	Low	7	2	8	6	4			
1374245_at	High	9	9	7	3	1	0.030	HL	6
	Low	3	4	8	12	2			
1374304_at	High	10	10	3	2	0	0.000	HL	2
	Low	2	2	7	13	2			
1375956_at	High	12	12	7	2	0	0.002	HL	2
	Low	3	4	9	10	2			
1375976_a_a t	High	8	7	2	5	2	0.016	HL	2
	Low	2	1	9	4	1			
1376611_at	High	11	6	5	2	0	0.006	HL	2
	Low	2	3	5	10	2			
1377137_at	High	13	8	5	3	0	0.005	HL	2
	Low	4	3	7	11	3			
1377902_a_a t	High	11	7	4	5	0	0.004	HL	2
	Low	2	3	8	11	4			
1379499_at	High	9	7	8	4	0	0.025	HL	6
	Low	3	4	7	11	4			
1379654_at	High	10	9	5	3	0	0.005	HL	2
	Low	6	1	7	9	4			
1382030_at	High	8	11	3	1	3	0.002	HLH	2
	Low	3	2	6	9	1			
1382783_at	High	7	11	3	2	0	0.006	HL	2
	Low	5	3	7	10	3			
1383251_at	High	11	6	5	3	1	0.015	HL	2
	Low	3	2	9	11	1			
1383953_at	High	14	7	5	2	0	0.000	HL	2
	Low	2	2	7	12	3			
1384029_at	High	10	7	8	0	0	0.001	HL	6
	Low	6	1	7	9	4			
1384257_at	High	11	9	6	2	1	0.028	HL	2
	Low	3	6	7	10	2			
1384378_at	High	13	8	6	4	0	0.016	HL	2
	Low	2	7	8	9	2			

1384523_at	High	11	9	5	2	1	0.006	HL	2
	Low	4	2	7	11	2			
1385006_at	High	3	5	10	9	0	0.013	LHL	2
	Low	7	9	1	6	2			
1385733_at	High	3	4	9	9	3	0.018	LH	2
	Low	13	5	6	4	0			
1385803_at	High	11	10	3	3	1	0.002	HL	2
	Low	5	0	8	9	1			
1386910_a_at	High	2	5	5	9	3	0.019	LH	0.7
	Low	8	3	10	3	0			
1388254_a_at	High	5	4	6	7	4	0.039	LH	6
	Low	9	9	8	2	0			
1388550_at	High	5	2	5	10	4	0.016	LH	2
	Low	7	11	5	5	0			
1389011_at	High	6	12	6	1	0	0.000	HL	2
	Low	4	1	8	12	4			
1389431_at	High	9	6	6	4	0	0.015	HL	6
	Low	1	4	5	10	3			
1389555_at	High	10	10	7	3	0	0.027	HL	6
	Low	4	4	9	7	4			
1390384_at	High	10	7	3	6	4	0.017	HLH	2
	Low	6	3	12	7	0			
1391078_at	High	12	7	4	4	0	0.005	HL	2
	Low	2	3	8	9	3			
1391491_a_at	High	12	5	5	2	4	0.000	HLH	2
	Low	2	3	8	13	0			
1393367_at	High	9	9	5	6	0	0.049	HL	2
	Low	4	3	8	7	4			
1393405_at	High	4	6	5	2	4	0.045	HLH	6
	Low	2	5	8	9	0			
1393798_at	High	1	2	12	11	0	0.000	LHL	2
	Low	9	6	4	3	4			
1393963_at	High	7	10	5	3	0	0.014	HL	2
	Low	5	3	9	10	4			
1394205_at	High	5	2	7	11	3	0.031	LH	2
	Low	11	8	5	6	0			
1395488_at	High	9	10	6	1	0	0.000	HL	2
	Low	6	1	6	11	4			
1395667_at	High	5	5	4	12	4	0.003	LH	6
	Low	6	7	10	1	0			

Table 9. Distribution of the number of experimental animals by levels of expressions of active genes and formaldehyde concentration for GO:0006281. Patterns of behavior of active genes: LH – monotonically increasing; HL – monotonically decreasing; LHL – convex; HLH – bent; C-complex. Genes determined to be active by both PS and Thomas et al. (2007) methods are shaded. For finding the pattern a statistical test is used (χ^2 test for proportions, $p<0.05$). The point of the first transition is established for each gene; it is defined as the smallest concentration at which changes in gene activity are determined (Fischer exact test, $p<0.05$).

3.5 Profiles of gene expression by formaldehyde concentration

The system effect of formaldehyde exposure is expressed in the pattern of changes in gene activity depending on the formaldehyde concentration. The reconstructions of all states of bio-objects are obtained for each GO-category. All parameters with High (Low) levels of values that have pre-determinicity degree no less than sufficient are obtained in the reconstructions. The complete set of reconstructions is structured by the concentration of formaldehyde: for each gene, a binary relationship "Level of values of gene – Concentration" is constructed (Table 9).

Each active gene is characterized by changes in levels of its values (level transitions) depending on formaldehyde concentration. Five types of transitions are introduced. These types help to understand system effects of exposure. Points of the first transition and types of transitions for all active genes in GO-categories are shown in Table 10. In these profiles the points of the first transition for large number of active genes is below 6 ppm.

GO-category	Point of the first transition				Transition type				
	0.7 ppm	2 ppm	6 ppm	15 ppm	LH	HL	LHL	HLH	C
GO:0004386	6	12	5	0	5	6	4	7	1
GO:0006281	3	36	14	0	9	32	4	7	1
GO:0006954	13	11	13	0	18	7	3	9	0
GO:0016604	2	14	3	0	8	8	1	2	0

Table 10. Number of active genes with characteristic behaviors for GO-categories.

This approach allows finding active genes and constructing profiles of their expression to establish the pattern of response to the formaldehyde concentration, when time is not considered.

3.6 Profiles of gene expressions by formaldehyde concentration accounting for the time

There is another parameter in the experiment, besides concentration. This parameter is the time point of observation. The concentration and the time are independent parameters of the experiment, but they become interconnected parameters in the system mechanisms that determine gene activity patterns. Actions of these parameters may be in different directions and patterns of their influence are complex. For finding the combined effect of two experimental parameters, it is required to establish significant differences of gene activity of exposed groups compared to the control group in each time point. In this problem, it is appropriate to use the whole scale, not just High and Low values. As a result, the solution would involve all bio-objects and all levels of parameters of their states.

Differences with the control group at each time point are found by using the Mann-Whitney criterion to the levels obtained by PS as the system knowledge. When difference is statistically significant for a gene at a time point, all bio-objects in the control group and that exposed group should show the same gene activity. This is verified by the scale of level aggregation (see Section 2.5). A gene is considered active, if the difference between aggregated levels of activity of that gene for the control and exposed groups is sufficiently large (not less than half of the scale diapason).

Application of this approach allows establishing of the following facts. There is a pattern in how genes in each GO-category reveal their activity at different time points, and the effect of the concentration compared to the effect of the time is insignificant (Fig. 7). The differential gene expression is mostly expressed in the first and last time points. At the lowest concentration (0.7 ppm), differential expressions are present for the most genes.

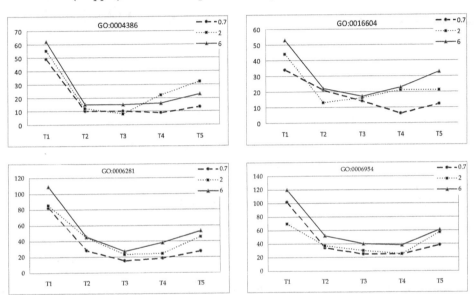

Fig. 7. Number of genes such that exposed groups (0.7 ppm, 2 ppm, 6 ppm) are different (according to the Mann-Whitney test) from the control group at each time point: x-axis – time points; y-axis – number of genes.

The procedure of transition to the aggregated levels for each gene is successful if all bio-objects at a time point are in one zone of the scale of level prevalence, i.e. express the same activity. For the simplified 3-item scale, this fact is reflected by Low, Medium, or High levels. When gene activity is different at the time point, the result of aggregation is not defined (0).

At the first time point (T1) the large number of genes in the control group has an undetermined level on the scale of level aggregation (Fig 8). The time parameter for this group introduces regularity in changes of gene activity. At the low formaldehyde concentration (0.07 ppm), at the first time point, almost every gene exhibited its characteristic level of activity, common for all bio-objects. In this time point of the experiment, the medium level of activity was the most common. At concentration 2 ppm, at the first time point, uncertainty of aggregated levels is lower than in the control group, but higher than in 0.7 ppm group. For 6 ppm concentration, the low level of activity is the most common. The distribution of the number of genes by aggregated levels, time points and concentrations varies considerably (Fig. 8).

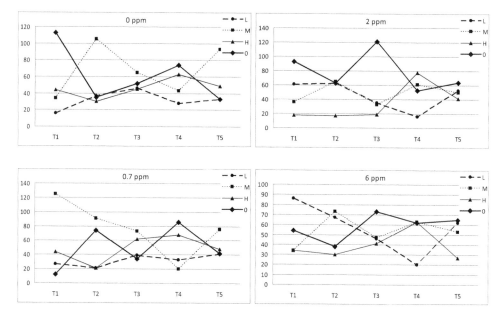

Fig. 8. Distribution of number of genes with aggregates values for concentration by time points (GO:0006281): x-axis – time points; y-axis – number of genes.

The following criteria were used for obtaining set of active genes accounting for both experimental parameters: (1) significant difference with control group and (2) sufficient difference between aggregated levels for the control group and at least one exposed group. Results of this method of determining gene activity accounting for both experimental parameters are compared with results of the method accounting only for the formaldehyde concentration in Table 11 (cf. Table 9). Genes belonging to a GO-category are distributed over six classes. Class 1 includes genes whose activity is determined by both methods and both methods resulted in the same point of the first transition. Class 2 includes genes whose activity is also determined by both methods, but the points of the first transition are different. Class 3 includes genes that are active only according to the second method. Class 4 includes genes active according to the first method, but only weakly active according to the second method. Class 5 contains genes such that according to the second method there is a difference with control group, but activity is weak (the difference between aggregated levels of the exposed and the control groups is not sufficient). Class 6 includes genes activity of which is not found by any of the two methods. Almost all genes in the GO-categories demonstrated activity caused by exposure when accounting for time. Degree of this activity could be measured.

The combined effect of both experimental parameters is illustrated with profiles of expression, obtained for different classes of genes. Profiles are unfolded in the time series for different formaldehyde concentration (Fig. 9). Probe 1383953_at belongs to class 1. Profiles of expression of this gene by time points are analogous for almost all concentrations of formaldehyde. Clear effect of changes in gene activity is revealed at 2 ppm. Probe

1368204_at belongs to class 2. The first approach found point of the first transition at 2 ppm, but for the second approach that point is at 0.7 ppm. Probe 1370172_at belongs to class 3. The time dependence of the gene expression profiles of the exposed groups are in anti-phase with the time dependence of the gene expression profile of the control group. Activity determined by the second method. Activity of probe 1391078_at from class 4 is determined by the second approach as weak. In all time points there are no sufficient differences with control group, however the weak activity for the 2 ppm concentration which is the point of the first transition determined by the first method is revealed. Probe 1395419_at belongs to

Gene classes	Number of genes in a class	Formaldehyde concentration			Distribution of active genes according to Thomas et al. (2007) in a class
		0.7 ppm	2 ppm	6 ppm	
GO:0004386					
1	13	3	9	1	8
2	4	2	2	0	2
3	43	14	19	10	14
4	6				1
5	47				7
6	8				2
GO:0006281					
1	17	2	9	6	11
2	18	0	16	2	7
3	68	27	7	34	11
4	18				7
5	68				8
6	15				0
GO:0006954					
1	15	7	4	4	7
2	12	2	5	5	4
3	108	42	33	33	8
4	10				2
5	108				12
6	28				2
GO:0016604					
1	11	2	7	2	6
2	6	0	5	1	2
3	41	13	9	19	10
4	2				1
5	52				18
6	10				2

Table 11. The distribution of all genes by their classes of activity. In the last column, intersection of genes determined by PS in certain class and active genes determined by Thomas et al. (2007) are shown.

class 5. The second approach determined difference in gene expression from the control for all exposed concentrations, but these differences are small. Neither the first, nor the second method determined probe 1367455_at as active.

In the problem of determining points of the first transition and type of transition, the time parameter is important, as both parameters of experiment influence activity complexly. Accounting for both parameters allows: to divide genes into classes of activity that characterize the form of revealing of combined effect of both parameters; to reveal larger number of active genes; and to reveal a substantial number of genes with small changes in their activity.

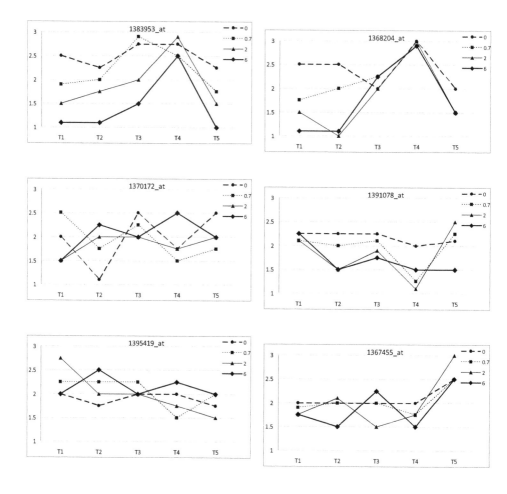

Fig. 9. Examples of profiles of gene expression for 6 classes of genes: x-axis – time points; y-axis – aggregated levels.

4. Conclusion

Physics of Open Systems overcomes complexity of bio-entities by understanding the nature of heterogeneity among them and using that understanding to create the reconstructions of their states. The reconstructions of states of bio-entities allow determination of levels of gene activity. This results in the profiles of gene activity. The reconstructions of states open the path to a deeper understanding of the mechanisms that determine levels of gene activity and determine the systematic responses of experimental animals to the formaldehyde exposure.

The data used in this article comes from the experiment described in Thomas et al. (2007). We considered an example of four GO-categories. For each active gene, we determined the point of the first transition, i.e. where the level of activity of the gene changes significantly (up or down). Our results indicate that the point of the first transition was most often found below 6 ppm, suggesting the absence of a threshold at 6 ppm. We conclude that there is a substantial gene activity below what had been proposed as a threshold of gene activity based on statistical BMD analysis (Thomas et al., 2007).

Some discussion about dose-response controversy is in order. A contentious issue in health risk assessment is whether or not effects observed at high doses in a bioassay can be extrapolated to low level of environmental exposures because MOAs may differ between high and low doses. Therefore, the issue of interest to us is to determine whether gene expression pattern is similar between high and low doses rather than finding only a subset of genes that may be responsible for the effects observed in bioassays. This issue is particularly important if the attempt has been made to use gene expression pattern to establish a threshold effect.

A number of genes from the 'DNA repair' GO category (GO:0006281), that is traditionally thought to be relevant to formaldehyde MOA (e.g. Thomas et al., 2007), were found active in our study in contrast to the Thomas et al. (2007) analysis (Table 9). Among these active genes in discrepancy with the analysis performed in the original study are: alpha 1 subunit of DNA directed polymerase (Gene symbol: Pola1 and probe ID:1376611_at), putative apurinic/apyrimidinic endonuclease 2 (RGD1565983, 1395667_at), APEX nuclease 1– a multifunctional DNA repair enzyme (Apex1, 1371217_at) and DNA non-homologous end-joining factor 1 (Nhej1, 1374245_at). Some of these enzymes are essential for various DNA repair processes. For example Nhej1 is an important component of non-homologous end-joining (NHEJ) repair of DNA double strand breaks (Buck et al., 2006, Ahnesorg et al., 2006, Tsai et al., 2007). Table 9 lists the active genes in 'DNA repair' GO category and characterizes them by the point of the first transition and type of change. Monotonic increase and monotonic decrease are labeled LH and HL respectively. Nhej1 and Pola1genes showed monotonic decrease with formaldehyde concentration, with Pola1 first transition at 2 ppm, and Nhej1 at 6 ppm (Table 9). Overall, 32 genes from 'DNA repair' category exhibit monotonic decrease and 25 of them have the first transition at a low, 2 ppm dose (Tables 9 and 10). Our results suggest that inhibition of key DNA repair proteins at transcriptional level might be an important component of formaldehyde genotoxicity at doses as low as 2 ppm. Formaldehyde inhibition of expression of proteins related to non-homologous end-joining (NHEJ) repair of DNA double strand breaks and base-excision repair (BER) of DNA adducts has been observed previously (Zhang et al., 2011). In particular, reduction of Ogg1, a key participant in BER, and Ku 70, which regulates NHEJ processes, was detected in cell culture exposed to 150 μM formaldehyde (Zhang et al., 2011). However it is difficult to relate the concentrations of formaldehyde used in these *in vitro* experiments to the doses used in the *in vivo* study for the present analysis.

Important benefit of application of PS methods to the genomics data is its ability to account for both parameters (exposure concentrations and time) of the experiment, something that simpler methods of analysis (e.g. Thomas et al., 2007) are not able to accomplish. The time of observation is a very important parameter for determining gene activity. Almost all genes in the four GO-categories demonstrated activity caused by exposure when accounting for time (Table 11).

Simple methods such as the one proposed by Thomas et al. (2007) cannot be expected to adequately explain the complexity of genomics data. Such simple methods may lead to an erroneous conclusion of a threshold effect that does not exist. More appropriate methods, like the one proposed in this article, are needed for a proper analysis of genomics data.

5. Acknowledgement

Research of authors from Saint-Petersburg State Polytechnic University was supported by ISTC grant number 3476, 2006-2011. The views expressed in this article are those of the authors and do not necessarily reflect the views or policies of the U.S. Environmental Protection Agency.

6. References

Ahnesorg, P., Smith, P. & Jackson, S.P. (2006). XLF interacts with the XRCC4-DNA ligase IV complex to promote DNA nonhomologous end-joining. *Cell*, Vol.124, No.2, pp. 301-313

Buck, D., Malivert, L., de Chasseval, R., Barraud, A., Fondanèche, M.C. & Sanal, O. (2006). Cernunnos, a novel nonhomologous end-joining factor, is mutated in human immunodeficiency with microcephaly. *Cell*, Vol.124, No.2, pp. 287-299

Conolly, R.B., Kimbell, J.S., Janszen, D., Schlosser, P.M., Kalisak, D., Preston, J., et al. (2004). Human respiratory tract cancer risks of inhaled formaldehyde: dose-response predictions derived from biologically motivated computational modeling of a combined rodent and human dataset. *Toxicological Sciences*, Vol.82, No.1, pp. 279–296

Conway, J.H. & Guy, R.K. (1996) *Farey Fractions and Ford Circles. The Book of Numbers*, Springer-Verlag, New York, NY

Crump KS. (1984). A new method for determining allowable daily intakes. *Fundamental Applications Toxicology*, Vol.4, No.5, pp. 854–871

Crump, K.S., Chen, C., Fox, J.F., van Landingham, C. & Subramaniam, R. (2008). Sensitivity analysis of biologicallymotivated model for formaldehyde-induced respiratory cancer in humans. *The Annals of Occupational Hygiene*, Vol.52, No.6, pp. 481-495

Hollander, M. & Wolfe, D. (1999). *Nonparametric statistical methods*, John Wiley and Sons, New York, NY

Kachanova, T. & Fomin, B. (1999). *Basis of Systemology of Phenomenal*, SPbGETU, ISBN 5-7629-0293-5, St.Petersburg, Russia

Kachanova, T. & Fomin, B. (2002). *Meta-technology of System Reconstruction*, SPbGETU, ISBN 5-7629-0439-3, St.Petersburg, Russia

Kachanova, T. & Fomin, B. (2003). *Technology of System Reconstruction*, Polytechnica, ISBN 5-7325-0772-8, St.Petersburg, Russia

Kachanova, T. & Fomin, B. (2009). *Introduction to the Language of Systems*, Nauka, ISBN 978-5-02-025360-5, St.Petersburg, Russia

Kachanova, T. & Fomin, B. (2010). Physics of Systems is a postcybernetic paradigm of systemology, *Proceedings of WMSCI 2010 14th World Multi-Conference on Systemics, Cybernetics and Informatics*, pp. 244-249, ISBN-13: 978-1-936338-00-9 (Volume III), Orlando, Florida, USA, June 29th - Jule 12nd, 2010

Kendall, M. (1970). *Rank correlation methods*, Charles Griffin, London, UK

Kerns, W., Pavkov, K., Donofrio, D., Gralla, E. & Swenberg, J. (1983). Carcinogenicity of formaldehyde in rats and mice after long-term inhalation exposure. *Cancer Research*, Vol.43, No.9, (September 1983), pp. 4382-4392

Monticello, T., Swenberg, J., Gross, E., Leininger, J., Kimbell, J., Seilkop, S., et al. (1996). Correlation of regional and nonlinear formaldehyde-induced nasal cancer with proliferating population of cells. *Cancer Research*, Vol.56, No.5, (March 1996), pp. 1012-1022

Saaty, T.L. (1980). *The Analytic Hierarchy Process: Planning, Priority Setting, Resource Allocation*, McGraw-Hill, New York, NY

Shannon, C.E. (1948). A mathematical theory of communication, *Bell System Technical Journal*, Vol.27, (July, October 1948), pp. 379-423 and 623-656

Thomas, R., Allen, B., Nong, A., Yang, L., Bermudez, E., Clewell, H., et al. (2007). A method to integrate benchmark dose estimates with genomic data to assess the functional effects of chemical exposure. *Toxicological Sciences*, Vol.98, No.1, (July 2007), pp. 240-248

Tsai, C.J., Kim, S.A. & Chu, G. (2007). Cernunnos/XLF promotes the ligation of mismatched and noncohesive DNA ends. *Proceedings of National Academy of Sciences of the USA*, Vol.104, No. 19, pp.7851-7856

U.S. Environmental Protection Agency. (2005). *Guidelines for Carcinogen Risk Assessment*. EPA/630/P-03/001F

U. S. Environmental Protection Agency. (2006). *Help Manual for Benchmark Dose Software - Version 1.4*. EPA/600/R-00/014F, http://www.epa.gov/ncea/bmds/

Yu, X., Griffith, W.C., Hanspers. K., Dillman. J.F. III, Ong, H., Vredevoogd, M.A., et al. (2006). A system-based approach to interpret dose- and time-dependent microarray data: Quantitative integration of gene ontology analysis for risk assessment. *Toxicological Sciences*, Vol.92, No.2, (August 2006), pp. 560-577

Zhang, R., Kang, K.A., Piao, M.J., Kim, K.C., Lee, N.H., You, H.J., et al. (2011). Triphlorethol-a improves the non-homologous end joining and base-excision repair capacity impaired by formaldehyde. *Journal of Toxicological and Environmental Health Part A*, Vol.74, No.12, pp. 811-821

7

Breast Cancer Prognostication and Risk Prediction in the Post-Genomic Era

Xi Zhao[1,2], Ole Christian Lingjærde[3,4] and Anne-Lise Børresen-Dale[1,2]
[1]Department of Genetics, Institute for Cancer Research, Oslo University Hospital,
The Norwegian Radium Hospital, Montebello,
[2]Institute of Clinical Medicine, University of Oslo,
[3]Biomedical Research Group, Department of Informatics, Faculty of Mathematics
and Natural Sciences, University of Oslo,
[4]Center for Cancer Biomedicine, University of Oslo,
Norway

1. Introduction

Today, breast cancer is appreciated as a group of molecularly distinct neoplastic disorders. Breast tumors are highly heterogeneous in pathology with respect to cell type and tissue origin. With the traditional diagnostic tools, patients with the same clinico-pathological parameters can have markedly different clinical courses. Individual tumors can frequently exhibit heterogeneous patterns of somatic mutations (Bamford et al. 2004, Stephens et al. 2009, Russnes et al. 2010) gene amplifications and deletions (Russnes et al. 2010), epigenetic profiles (Rønneberg et al. 2010), and gene expression portraits (Perou et al. 2000). Efforts to significantly impact cancer patient outcomes will require the development of robust strategies to subdivide such heterogeneous panels of cancers into biologically and clinically homogenous subgroups, for the purposes of personalizing treatment protocols and identifying optimal drug targets.

In this chapter, by reviewing published, as well as unpublished work, we outline the application of microarray expression profiling in breast cancer risk assessment; highlight the strategies of developing molecular classifiers and integrative strategies to improve risk stratification for breast cancer patients. We also discuss the limitations of the "first-generation" expression profiling as well as further methodologies.

2. Prognostication and risk prediction in breast cancer

Breast cancer is indeed a heterogeneous disease with large variation in clinical behavior. There exist a variety of prognostic factors associated with patient survival (such as susceptibility to metastasize) and some predictive markers (which can aid selection of relevant systemic therapy) for management of the breast cancer patient.

2.1 Clinico-pathological prognostic and predictive markers

Traditionally, the treatment decision for breast cancer patients is largely based on a number of histo-pathological features including tumor size, axillary lymph node status, histological grade, TNM staging (Tumor size, regional lymph Nodes, distant Metastasis) and receptor status.

Tumor size

The size of a tumor is an established prognosis marker used in the clinic (Koscielny et al. 1984, Rosen et al. 1989, Carter et al. 1989, Page 1991). Tumors under 2 cm (T1) in diameter have a low risk of metastasis; tumors of 2-5 cm (T2) have a high risk of metastasis; tumors over 5 cm (T3) have a very high risk of metastasis. Tumor size carries independent prognosis value; both the axillary lymph node status and histological grade are related to tumor size (Rosen et al. 1989, Carter et al. 1989, Weigelt et al. 2005).

Axillary lymph node status

The axillary lymph node status (Carter et al. 1989, Rosen et al. 1989, Page 1991) is another established marker that has been used in clinic setting to characterize the risk of developing metastatic breast cancer. The presence of cancer cells in the lymph nodes increases the risk of metastatic breast cancer. The presence of over four lymph-node metastases is associated with very high metastatic risk.

Histological grade

Histological grade (Scarff et al. 1968) is a well-known histo-pathological parameter routinely used in the clinic to describe the similarity of breast cancer cells to normal breast tissue, and classify the cancer into well differentiated (low grade: Histological grade 1), moderately differentiated (intermediate grade: Histological grade 2), and poorly differentiated (high grade: Histological grade 3), reflecting progressively less normal appearing cells that have a worsening prognosis.

TNM staging

The TNM classification of malignant tumors (TNM) uses the size of the primary tumor (T), its nodal involvement (N), and the presence of distant metastases (M) to classify the progression of cancer into stage I to stage IV. Breast cancers classified as stage I are small and localized tumors, generally have good prognosis, while stage IV tumors are the most advanced and metastatic with poor prognosis. The staging system classifies breast tumors into groups with different prognosis profiles. Carcinoma *in situ* is indicated as stage 0 in the TNM classification. The stage of a cancer is one of the most important factors in determining prognosis and treatment options.

Receptor status

Protein expression of three receptors in breast cancer cells are routinely used in the clinic: estrogen receptor (ER), progesterone receptor (PgR) and Human Epidermal growth factor Receptor 2 (HER2; also known as HER2/neu, ErbB-2 or ERBB2). When treated with tamoxifen, breast cancer patients with tumors that are ER+ and/or PR+ have lower risks of mortality after their diagnosis compared to women with ER- and/or PgR-negative disease (Fisher et al. 1988). Determination the presence of the estrogen receptor is critical for the selection of the patients who could benefit form endocrine treatment (e.g. tamoxifen). Immunohistochemical (IHC) analysis is widely used to measure ER and PgR protein expression. HER2 is a protein involved in regulation of cellular growth giving higher aggressiveness in breast cancers. HER2+ breast cancer had a worse prognosis (Slamon et al. 1989, Sotiriou and Pusztai 2009). Cells with none of these receptors are called triple negative. This type of breast cancer is clinically characterized as more aggressive and less responsive to standard treatment and associated with poorer overall patient survival (Dent et al. 2007, Chustecka 2007).

Some of the above traditional variables are combined into prognostic models (such as Adjuvant Online! and Nottingham Prognostic Index) for treatment decision-making about adjuvant systemic treatment of patients with early breast cancer.

Adjuvant Online! model

Adjuvant! Online (Ravdin et al. 2001) is a computer based model using patient age, comorbidity level, ER status, tumor grade, tumor size and number of positive lymph nodes to predict breast cancer specific mortality and recurrence risk, as well as the benefit of adjuvant therapy for women with early-stage breast cancer. Because Adjuvant! was directly derived from mortality data and because details of local therapy (surgery and initial radiation) can strongly influence local relapse rates more so than mortality, Adjuvant!'s estimates of mortality are more firmly based than those for relapse. Breast cancer outcome estimates made by Adjuvant! are for "patients who have unilateral, unicentric, invasive adenocarcinoma of the breast, who have undergone definitive primary breast surgery and axillary node staging, and who have no evidence of metastatic or known residual disease; no evidence of T4 features (extension to skin or chest wall); no evidence of inflammatory breast cancer. If they have had breast conserving therapy there should be plans for them to receive radiation therapy. They should not yet have received systemic therapy (neoadjuvant therapy), or radiation prior to their surgical staging." (Adjuvant! Breast Cancer Help Files http://www.adjuvantonline.com/breastnew.jsp Accessed on December 15, 2011).

Nottingham Prognostic Index

The Nottingham prognostic index (NPI) (Haybittle et al. 1982) is used to determine prognosis following surgery for breast cancer by integrating the size of the lesion; the number of involved lymph nodes; and the grade of the tumor. A prognostic index < 3.4 implies a good prognosis, in the range of [3.4, 5.4] a moderately good prognosis and > 5.4 a poor prognosis. It was established by the long-term follow-up in a dedicated breast unit of patients who did not receive adjuvant therapy, had a standard management.

2.2 Gene expression profiling approaches

Although the current diagnostic tools are valuable, breast cancer is still one of the most frequent cause of cancer death worldwide (Garcia et al. 2007). There is clearly a need for improved diagnostic tools that are highly sensitive and specific to stratify patients and predict risk of recurrence and therapeutic sensitivities on a continuous scale to aid individualized decision making for the treatment.

Microarrays where expression profiling of thousands of messenger RNA transcripts takes place in a single experiment have been evolving in the past decade to become an established approach in biological research. Genome-wide expression profiling has led to a better stratification of breast cancer and has been useful for outcome prediction.

2.2.1 Microarrays

Microarray technology allows genome-wide interrogation of mRNA expression by hybridization of labeled RNA (or cDNA) to complementary sequences that are arrayed on a chip. After washing off the excess, the array is processed by a laser scanner to produce an image of differential signal intensities. The intensity of each probe can then be linked to the RNA abundance of the corresponding gene.

The basic procedure in an experiment involves the isolation of RNA or messenger RNA (mRNA) from appropriate biological samples, reverse transcription of mRNA into complementary DNA (cDNA) and hybridization of the fluorescence-labeled cDNA to the microarray. After washing off the excess, the array is processed by a laser scanner to produce an image of differential signal intensities. Dual-channel microarrays are typically hybridized with cDNA prepared from test (e.g. tumor) and reference (e.g. normal). It provides a relative measurement level for the corresponding RNA molecule. The one-channel arrays provide intensity for each probe (or probe set) indicating a relative level of hybridization.

Microarray platforms can be classified with respect to their manufacturing (spotted cDNA or oligonucleotide) and hybridization quantification (single or dual-channel). In spotted microarrays, the probes are synthesized prior to deposition on the array surface and are then spotted onto the chip. A common approach utilizes an array of fine pins or needles controlled by a robotic arm that is dipped into wells containing DNA probes and then depositing each probe at specific locations on the array surface. In oligonucleotide microarrays, the probes are short DNA sequences designed to match parts of the sequence of known or predicted gene coding regions. Oligonucleotide arrays are produced by chemically synthesizing short oligonucleotide sequences directly onto the array surface. Sequences may be longer (60-mer probes such as the Agilent Design) or shorter (25-mer probes produced by Affymetrix). Longer probes are more specific to individual target genes, and shorter probes may be spotted in higher density across the array and are cheaper to manufacture. Other microarray platforms, such as Illumina bead-based platforms (San Diego, CA, USA), use microscopic beads, instead of the large solid support.

In single-channel microarrays, a single mRNA source is hybridized on a chip and comparison of RNA levels between samples is made *in silico* in a post-processing phase of the experiment. In dual-channel microarrays, two mRNA sources are used, each labeled with different fluors. The second mRNA source is usually either a common reference against which all samples in an experiment are compared to, or a sample coming from a tissue under an alternative condition (e.g. tumor versus normal).

2.2.2 Strategies to develop gene-expression prognostic signatures

In general, strategies to develop a gene-expression prognostic signature from microarray data include the so-called *"top-down"* and *"bottom-up"* approaches (Sotiriou and Pusztai 2009). In the first strategy, identification of genes associated with prognosis is carried out in a supervised fashion guided by known clinical outcomes without any *a priori* biologic assumption (van 't Veer et al. 2002, Wang et al. 2005), while in the bottom-up discovery approach, genes associated with a specific biologic phenotype or a deregulated molecular pathway are first identified and then subsequently correlated with the clinical outcome

(Chang et al. 2005, Chi et al. 2006). In addition, a *candidate-gene* approach, utilized in development of Oncotype DX® (Paik et al. 2004) is based on data from quantitative reverse-transcriptase-polymerase chain reaction (Q-RT-PCR); the technique selects genes of interest on the basis of existing biologic knowledge which are then combined into a multivariate predictive model.

In high-throughput molecular profiling, the number of genes is typically much larger than the number of samples ($p>>n$), which would run into the phenomenon commonly referred to as the curse of dimensionality (Bellman 1961). Feature selection and dimension reduction often become key steps in the microarray data analysis. However, feature selection in microarray data is a nontrivial task due to high dimensionality, correlation between variables (features) and sometimes high level of noise. Below, we outline the common strategies used in gene expression data for signature construction, including feature selection, unsupervised analysis and supervised learning (Figure 1). See Hastie et al. (2001) for a review of statistical learning methods for high-dimensional problems.

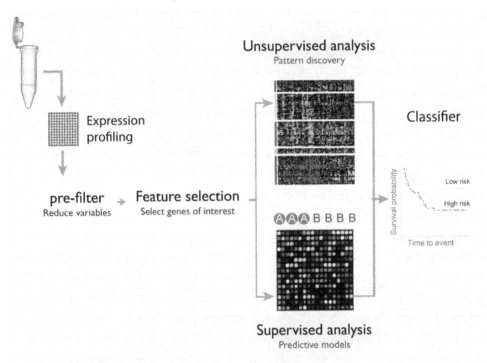

Fig. 1. Analytic pipeline for the development of a Gene-Expression Prognostic Signature.

Feature selection

Feature selection is different from quality filtering, where the reduction of the number of genes are carried out purely based on the quality of the measurement (such as signal-to-noise ratio, variance) without any information related to the outcome. A commonly used strategy for feature selection is to rank the genes (features) by their relevance to the outcome of interest and then apply a cut-off to select the most interesting genes. Choice of model and statistical test depends on the characteristics of the outcome measurement, including whether it is quantitative (e.g. time to event) or categorical (e.g. tumor versus normal). Significance analysis of microarrays or SAM (Tusher et al. 2001) is one of the widest used methods in identifying differentially expressed genes in data arising from microarray experiments. It is a t-statistics variant that compares group means, adapted to a high-dimensional setting. Another popular approach is the empirical Bayes methods in the context of linear models (Smyth 2004). The empirical Bayes, SAM and other shrinkage methods (Smyth et al. 2005) are used to borrow information across genes to make the inferences stable when the number of arrays is small.

While the above filter methods assess the relevance of features, it ignores the effects of the selected feature subset on the accuracy of the model. The subset selection strategies assess subsets of features according to their relevance for a given model. These methods conduct a search for a good subset using the model itself as part of the evaluation function (e.g. stepwise regression by optimizing criteria such as AIC, BIC, Mallow's C_p, etc). Subset selection can also be achieved by cross-validation, where the samples are first split into $k > 1$ groups (or "folds") of roughly equal size. Suppose the goodness-of-fit is expressed by a loss function (which in the case of a likelihood based method would be minus the log of the likelihood). Then, for each model (variable subset) to be assessed, a cross-validation score is calculated by fitting the model to all samples except those in the j'th fold (j = 1, 2, ..., k), computing the loss function on the remaining fold, and adding together all the contributions. The model with the smallest cross-validation score is then selected.

In addition, methods embedded with internal variable selection (e.g. LASSO, PAM and decision tree) have also become popular tools for selecting a set of potential gene candidates from high-dimensional expression data. More complex model selection procedures such as double-loop k-fold cross-validation are sometimes used to determine several model parameters simultaneously.

Unsupervised pattern discovery

Unsupervised analyses are used to describe how the data are organized and find structures in the data. We only observe the features and do not use measurements of the outcome. Unsupervised methods such as hierarchical clustering, K-means clustering and self-organizing maps make it possible to identify groups of patients with similar gene expressions or groups of genes with similar expression pattern (co-expression gene cluster). The resulting patient groups are subsequently correlated with the clinical outcome as well as clinico-pathological parameters to assess the clinical relevance of the input gene markers.

Hierarchical clustering is an agglomerative approach in which single expression profiles are joined to form groups, which are further joined until the process has been carried to completion, forming a single hierarchical tree. There are several variations on hierarchical clustering that differ in how distances are measured between pairs of observations (distance metric) and between clusters (linkage criteria) as they are constructed. Hierarchical clustering is often criticized for giving ambiguous results because of sensitivity to data perturbation or clustering techniques used. The challenge is to select the algorithms appropriately so that the data is sensibly partitioned. Criteria such as the Gap statistic (Tibshirani et al. 2001), silhouette (Rousseeuw 1987), and bootstrap resampling (Suzuki and

Shimodaira 2004) are used to decide the optimal number, the quality and the reproducibility of the clusters, respectively. Often, external information about tumor characteristics (e.g. *TP53* mutation status, histological subtype, estrogen receptor status, etc) can be useful to evaluate to what extent the resulting tumor clusters fit with the existing prior knowledge.

Another commonly used unsupervised method is principal component analysis (PCA). It is a dimension reduction technique that produces linear combinations of the original variables to generate principal components (PCs) that are a set of uncorrelated variables. The first PC captures the highest variability presented in the data. PCA is useful for reduction of dimensionality by focusing on a few top principal components. Outliers can dominate the results of a principal components analysis.

The "*unsupervised*" approach aims at identifying subgroups of patients with similar gene expression pattern. The unsupervised learning process is not guided by any *a priori* biologic knowledge or clinical outcomes. In the "*supervised*" approach, markers associated with the outcome variable are identified. Validation (e.g. on an independent data set or using cross-validation procedure) is vital in the supervised learning process.

Supervised learning strategies

A supervised analysis aims to find a statistical relationship between input data (e.g. gene expressions) and output (e.g. response to a treatment or the survival of a patient). Supervised learning strategies can be further labeled according to whether outcome measurements are quantitative (regression) or qualitative (classification), as well as by whether models are designed to describe a current condition or predict future outcome based on a set of features (e.g. gene expression). A variety of models are available for regression and classification, respectively. Rather than elaborating each of these methods, we focus on the *regularization* approaches as the general remedy for the high-dimensionality in gene expression data.

When the number of explanatory variables genes (p) is large and even exceeds the number of individuals n used for training of the model, the fitted model typically performs well on the training data, but poorly on new observations. This is commonly referred to as overfitting and is a major concern in statistical analysis of high-dimensional data. In addition, a high degree of collinearity among the variables is likely to emerge, thereby leading to a situation in which the estimated regression coefficients may change substantially, even after slight perturbations of the training data.

In a linear model, dimension reduction techniques and penalized regression are the strategies to control and stabilize the variance of the estimates and further achieve better prediction rules. The primary goal in the penalized or regularized methods is to shrink the regression coefficients vector away from the ordinary least squares solution (in regression setting) and achieve improved the predictive performance through a bias-variance trade-off. Some widely used regression regularization methods such as ridge regression, partial least squares and principle components regression were compared in the studies by Frank and Friedman in 1993 (Frank and Friedman 1993) and Lingjærde and Christophersen in 2000 (Lingjærde and Christophersen 2000) . In Cox-ridge regression, the coefficients are estimated by maximization of the L2-penalized partial log-likelihood (using the Newton-Raphson procedure):

$$l_\lambda(\beta) = l(\beta) - \frac{1}{2}\lambda \sum_{i=1}^{p} \beta_i^2$$

where the first term is the partial log-likelihood and the second term is a penalty term in the form of a scaled L2 norm of the model coefficients (Verweij and Van Houwelingen 1994). Here, $\lambda > 0$ is a tunable penalty parameter that controls how much weight to put on the penalty function. The penalty parameter can be determined by the leave-one-out cross validation procedure proposed by Verweij and van Houwelingen (Verweij and Van Houwelingen 1993). Similar to ridge yet different, the lasso (Tibshirani 1996) is a penalized least squares method that imposes an L1 penalty on the regression coefficients. While ridge regression keeps all the predictors in the model, the lasso does both continuous shrinkage and automatic variable selection simultaneously. However, lasso is indifferent on the choice among a group of covariates that are strongly correlated. The elastic net penalty (Zou and Hastie 2005) was introduced as a compromise between ridge and lasso. The elastic-net simultaneously does automatic variable selection like the lasso and continuous shrinkage on the coefficients of correlated variables like ridge.

In a comparative study of survival prediction performance using microarray data (Bøvelstad et al. 2007), it has been found that Cox-ridge regression often outperforms other common regularization techniques for Cox regression, such as principal components regression, supervised principal components regression, partial least squares regression and the lasso.

Other supervised learning techniques, such as ensemble learning strategies (e.g. bagging, boosting and random forest) have also been applied to gene expression data analysis. The idea is to build a prediction model by combining the strengths of a number of weak learners. Refer to Hastie et al. (Hastie et al. 2001) for overview on a comprehensive collection of statistical learning methods.

2.2.3 Established gene signatures

Some of the established gene signatures with potential clinical usage are reviewed below. This review covers Intrinsic subtypes (Perou et al. 2000, Sørlie et al. 2001, Sørlie et al. 2003, Parker et al. 2009), MammaPrint® (van 't Veer et al. 2002), Wound-Response (Chang et al. 2004, Chang et al. 2005), 76-gene (Wang et al. 2005), Genomic Grade Index (Sotiriou et al. 2006), Oncotype DX® (Paik et al. 2004) and Hypoxia (Chi et al. 2006). For each of the gene signatures, we briefly describe the development procedures, the clinical characteristics for the targeted cohorts as originally intended (Table 1) and the critical requirements that are signature-specific for appropriate usage.

Expression-based molecular subtypes

The initial "intrinsic gene set" was found by searching genes that showed little variance within tumor samples (i.e., before and after neoadjuvant chemotherapy pairs), but high variance across different tumors (Perou et al. 2000). The signature that comprised the 496 intrinsic genes was further developed by unsupervised classifications that were based on clustering algorithms. The intrinsic signature was then used to classify breast tumors into five biological subgroups (luminal A, luminal B, HER2-enriched, basal-like, and normal-like) that show distinct clinical implications (Perou et al. 2000). There exist a couple of variants with different numbers of genes in the intrinsic gene set in subsequent publications (Sørlie et al. 2001, Sørlie et al. 2003, Hu et al. 2006, Perreard et al. 2006).

Signature	Predicted phenotype / Endpoint	Training Cohort	Validation Cohort
Intrinsic	Subtypes	Locally advanced BC	Consecutive BC
PAM50	Subtypes	Consecutive BC[1]	Consecutive BC
	5-year relapse	Node–	Node– & +
70gene	5 year distant metastasis	Node–	Node– & +
76gene	5 year distant metastasis	Node–	Node–
GGI	HG1- or HG3-like in HG2	ER+	Consecutive BC
WR	Active or Quiescent CSR	Representative BC[2]	Representative BC
	Population based prognosis		Consecutive BC
Hypoxia	Hypoxic or Non-hypoxic	Representative BC	Representative BC
RS	10 year distant metastasis	Tamoxifen-treated; ER+; Node–	Tamoxifen-treated; ER+; Node– & Node+

Table 1. Characteristics of the studied gene signatures and their clinically relevant breast cancer cohorts.

The molecular subtypes have profound impact in unveiling heterogeneities in breast cancers. The presence of distinct molecular entities suggests the existence of multiple "cells of origin"(Prat and Perou 2009). There has been a shift in how the subtypes are defined over time, such as including more proliferation-associated genes (Hu et al. 2006, Parker et al. 2009). This may partially explain the discordance between PAM50 and Intrinsic, with respect to LumA and LumB classification. In our study (Zhao et al. Unpublished), we compared the subtype classification between Intrinsic (Perou et al. 2000) and PAM50 (Parker et al. 2009) on a large breast cancer dataset (van Vliet et al. 2008) (n = 947). Overall, subtype assignments of the signatures were moderately correlated (Cohen's kappa, $\kappa = 0.54$) (Cohen 1960). Noticeably, nearly half of the LumA tumors by Intrinsic were assigned as LumB by PAM50, while the two signatures appeared to highly agree on classification of basal-like subtype tumors. Indeed, basal-like was the most concordant subtype with a Pearson correlation of 0.94 between Intrinsic and PAM50, followed by normal-like (0.85), LumA (0.68), LumB (0.55) and Her2-enriched (0.42). More specifically, basal-like was the most distinctly classified subtype across these two signatures, as only those samples for which the correlation to basal-centroid by Intrinsic was slightly larger than the second highest centroid correlation showed inconsistent calls by PAM50.

As previously pointed out (Sørlie et al. 2010), an important issue for the molecular subtyping of breast cancers is the need for a clear definition of the molecular subtypes of breast cancer and standardized analytical methods to identify them. Until a consistent taxonomy is established, it is expected for inconsistent results when comparing assignments by various approaches that do not comprise the same entities.

70-gene signature

The 70-gene prognosis profile or MammaPrint® (Agendia, Amsterdam, The Netherlands) (van 't Veer et al. 2002) has been trained on a cohort of *lymph-node-negative* patients:

---

[1] *Consecutive BC*: heterogeneous breast cancer cohort with consecutive clinical parameter distribution as reflected in the whole population of this disease.

[2] *Representative BC*: breast cancer dataset at hand carries representative features that are associated with a certain breast cancer subpopulation.

expression of a set of 70 prognostic markers that was identified in a "supervised" fashion based on their ability to predict freedom from tumor metastasis (favorable prognosis) over a five-year period in the same dataset. It was validated subsequently on NKI295, a larger cohort consisting both node negative and positive patients (van de Vijver et al. 2002) and another validation study (Mook et al. 2008) was done on cohorts of 241 patients with 1-3 positive lymph nodes. Despite the fact that part of the validation set in the original retrospective validation study (van de Vijver et al. 2002) was overlapped with the training set of the signature (van 't Veer et al. 2002), the 70-gene signature has been validated in the independent cohort by the TRANSBIG consortium (Buyse et al. 2006). Espinosa *et al.* (Espinosa et al. 2005) reproduced with quantitative reverse-transcriptase-polymerase chain reaction (Q-RT-PCR) the results obtained with a 70-gene expression profile.

The gene signature classifies patient into good or bad prognostic group by the average profile of previously determined 70 genes in tumors from patients with a good prognosis. A patient with a correlation coefficient of more than 0.4 was then assigned to the group with a good-prognosis signature and all other patients were assigned to the group with a poor-prognosis signature. The threshold was set to achieve a 10 percent rate of false negative results in the 78 tumors in the previous study (van 't Veer et al. 2002).

76-gene signature

The 76-gene signature (Veridex) (Wang et al. 2005, Foekens et al. 2006, Desmedt et al. 2007a) is designed to predict distant metastasis within five years for lymph-node-negative breast cancer patients. It was original developed based on 286 lymph-node-negative breast cancer patients (Wang et al. 2005) and validated on an independent multicentric population of 180 untreated N- breast cancer patients (Foekens et al. 2006) and another gene expression study of 198 node-negative breast cancer patients (Desmedt et al. 2007a) from the same Affymetrix U133a platform as in the original study (Wang et al. 2005).

In the 76-gene signature (Wang et al. 2005), a relapse score is calculated for ER+ and ER- samples using sum of the weighted log2-gene-expression of the 60 genes and 16 genes, respectively:

$$\sum_{i=1}^{60} w_i x_i \text{ (for ER positive sample)}$$

$$\sum_{j=1}^{16} u_j y_j \text{ (for ER negative sample)}$$

where i and j indicate markers for ER positive and ER negative group, respectively; w_i and u_j are the standardized Cox regression coefficients for ER positive and ER negative markers, respectively; x_i and y_j are the expression values of ER positive and ER negative markers, respectively.

Intuitively, the pre-derived constants in the relapse model (Wang et al. 2005) are likely platform dependent. Additionally, we observed that the 76-gene signature was unable to identify any Desmedt sample (Desmedt et al. 2007a) with good prognosis when applied on RMA- instead of MAS5-normalized data. The discrepancies suggested that the risk cutoffs and possibly its original gene weights in the algorithm are sensitive to the data scale (Zhao et al. Unpublished).

Genomic Grade Index

The Genomic Grade Index (GGI) is a 97-gene measure of histologic tumor grade. The GGI was able to reclassify patients with histologic grade 2 tumors into two groups with distinct clinical outcomes similar to those of histologic grade 1 and 3, respectively (Sotiriou et al. 2006).

The Genomic Grade Index signature contains 128 Affymetix probes (representing 97 genes), of which 112 probes were with increased expression in histologic grade 3 tumors; and the remaining 16 probes with increased expression in histologic grade 1 tumors. The expressions of the 97 grade associated genes were further combined into the genomic grade index (GGI) by:

$$\sum_{j \in G_3} x_j - \sum_{j \in G_1} x_j$$

where x_j is the expression of either a grade 1 marker or grade 3 marker. The raw GGI scores were further scaled so that the mean of the GGI scores of histologic grade 1 tumors was -1 and that of histologic grade 3 tumors was $+1$:

$$GGI = scale(\sum_{j \in G_3} x_j - \sum_{j \in G_1} x_j - offset)$$

High GGI is associated with decreased relapse-free survival in both untreated and tamoxifen-treated patients (Loi et al. 2007). In the original publication (Sotiriou et al. 2006) the GGI signature was proposed to classify histologic grade 2 samples (or samples neither HG1 nor HG3) into "HG1-like" & "HG3-like". Tumors with a negative GGI score were classified as "HG1-like"; 0 or a positive GGI score put a tumor into "HG3-like" category. In the subsequent study (Haibe-Kains et al. 2008a), the authors dichotomized the raw GGI into "low-risk" and "high-risk" group based on 33% quartile in two different populations, VDX and TRANSBIG, respectively: the third of the patients having the lowest GGI scores being defined as low-risk and the remaining patients as high-risk. The population based prognostic strategy for GGI signature particularly requires that the samples are a good representative of the population of breast cancer with consecutive clinical parameter distribution.

GGI has a standardization procedure using the information of histological grade so that the mean of the GGI scores of histologic grade 1 tumors was -1 and that of histologic grade 3 tumors was +1, which is likely to increase its robustness when transferred to another array-based expression dataset (Zhao et al. Unpublished).

Wound response

The wound response or core serum response (CSR) gene signature (Chang et al. 2004) was derived from the transcriptional response of normal fibroblasts to serum in cell culture. It has been shown to improve the risk stratification of early breast cancer over that provided by standard clinic pathological features, in that the development of distant metastases is more likely among patients whose breast cancers have activated pathways for matrix remodeling, cell motility, and angiogenesis than among those whose cancers do not. The signature classifies tumors into two classes (*Activated* vs. *Quiescent*) through a centroid, which was built from the averaged fibroblast serum-induced expression pattern of the CSR genes (Chang et al. 2004, Chang et al. 2005).

Hypoxia signature

The epithelial hypoxia signature (Chi et al. 2006) consists of genes (253 image clones) that were consistently induced by hypoxia in cultured epithelial cells (HMECs and RPTECs). The 253 image clones were mapped to 168 Unigene clusters in the study (Chi et al. 2006). A "hypoxia score" was computed for a patient by averaging expression levels for the hypoxia response genes. Patients were assigned into high or low hypoxia response group by a cutoff hypoxia-score at zero (Nuyten et al. 2008). A positive score indicates *hypoxic* and non-positive score indicates *non-hypoxic*. Using published data sets, the authors found that the "high hypoxia response" group tends to be higher grade, and more likely to have p53 and oestrogen receptor deficiencies, and, most importantly, a significant association with a poorer prognosis in breast and ovarian cancer.

Oncotype DX®

Oncotype DX® (Genomic Health Inc., Redwood City, CA) (Paik et al. 2004) or the 21-gene-recurrence-score signature was developed from quantitative reverse transcription-polymerase chain reaction (Q-RT-PCR) assay to quantify the likelihood of distant recurrence at 10 years in adjuvant-tamoxifen-treated patients and further spare patients from adjuvant chemotherapy, in both node-negative (Paik et al. 2004) and node-positive disease(Albain et al. 2010). It includes 16 cancer-related genes that can be grouped into five different biological domains – proliferation, HER2 signaling, ER signaling, invasion and other – along with five reference genes. The linear combination of scores from these biological groups was computed and scaled into a Recurrence Score (RS), which is used to classifier a patient into categories of high risk (RS≥31), intermediate risk (18≤RS<31), and low risk of recurrence (RS<18).

Applying Oncotype DX® to a microarray-based dataset is not straightforward, which has often been underappreciated in existing studies (Fan et al. 2006, Loi et al. 2007). In Oncotype DX®, reference-normalized expression measurements ranged from 0 to 15, where one unit increase reflects approximately a 2-fold increase in RNA. The exact quantifications are hard to draw in the microarray-based measurements. We emphasize that only a pseudo RS based on the Oncotype DX® algorithm can be computed from microarray-based datasets.

Applicability of individual gene signatures

Translating the expression-based gene signatures to a new dataset is complicated by the heterogeneities derived from using several microarray, the differences of data processing procedures and the clinical uniqueness of each studied cohort.

We grouped the above gene signatures into two broad categories based on their associated approaches of summarizing expression values: *centroid-based* (Intrinsic, PAM50, 70-gene and WR) and *weighted average gene expression predictors* (76-gene, GGI, RS and Hypoxia).

For the 76-gene signature, the pre-derived constants in the relapse model are likely platform dependent. Ideally, applying this signature to a new dataset, one should follow the same protocol using the same platform with the same normalization procedure as in the original studies (Wang et al. 2005, Desmedt et al. 2007a). The Oncotype DX® (RS), another signature based on weighted sum method, also has potential issues related to the data scale in computing the recurrence score. Furthermore, the differences between the microarray and PCR technologies make the recurrence scores estimated from microarray experiments less optimal. GGI shares similarities with the 76-gene signature and Oncotype DX® in constructing risk estimation from gene expression pattern. However, GGI has a unique standardization procedure incorporating the information of histological grade, which likely increases its robustness when transferred to different microarray platforms. Generally, when the distribution of risk scores depends on platform and normalization procedure, as we found with some signatures, cutoffs for risk group assignment need to be recalibrated. The population-based strategy in which a fixed proportion of the population was assigned to each risk group is more general and applicable for a study with pure prognosis purpose on the new cohort. However, it particularly requires the samples to be representative of the population of breast cancer.

A previous study concluded that complex models are not better predictors of prognosis than simpler ones derived from gene expression studies (Haibe-Kains et al. 2008b). In general, we believe that successful models should be constructed in a robust way to tolerate cross-platform differences. This may explain why methods based on centroid correlations (such as subtype signatures and the 70-gene) or methods that transform the data into an invariant scale before computing the risk scores (such as GGI), have more consistent performances. We suspect that the weighted average fashion is more sensitive to the data scale and the issue of missing signature gene(s) in the data at hand.

2.3 Limitations of the "first-generation" expression profiling

Gene expression profiling has opened a door for personalized medicine. However, the "first-generation" gene signatures may offer no more than a snapshot of a tumor's gene expression profile that is most relevant for only a particular point in time. Meanwhile, tumor development is essentially Darwinian and tumor heterogeneity is dynamic as selective pressures change during the metastatic process. The complex structural network of the tumor system and the vital interactions of tumor cells with stromal and immune cells highlight the need for a cellular systems biology approach to cancer diagnostics, which combines multiplexed biomarker panels with informatics tools to produce a systemic readout relevant to patient prognosis. Comprehensive genomic analysis of tumor subpopulations of the host patient is likely the best way to effectively use gene signatures from both patient and tumor, so that treatment plans can be optimized.

2.3.1 Influence of time and ER status on gene signatures in breast cancer survival prediction

In Zhao et al. (Zhao et al. Unpublished), we assessed several prognostic gene signatures that have received the greatest interest and been validated in multiple studies. These include the *Intrinsic signature* (Perou et al. 1999, Perou et al. 2000, Sørlie et al. 2001, Sørlie et al. 2003), *PAM50* (Parker et al. 2009), 70-gene profile or MammaPrint® (Agendia, Amsterdam, The

Netherlands) (van 't Veer et al. 2002, van de Vijver et al. 2002, Mook et al. 2008, Buyse et al. 2006, Espinosa et al. 2005), 76-gene signature (Wang et al. 2005, Foekens et al. 2006, Desmedt et al. 2007a), Genomic Grade Index (GGI) (Sotiriou et al. 2006, Loi et al. 2007), wound response (WR) signature (Chang et al. 2004, Chang et al. 2005), hypoxia signature (Chi et al. 2006, Nuyten et al. 2008) and 21-gene-recurrence-score (RS) or Oncotype DX® (Genomic Health Inc., Redwood City, CA) (Paik et al. 2004).

The eight signatures were applied on an expression dataset (van Vliet et al. 2008) (n = 947) pooled from six published breast cancer datasets (Loi et al. 2007, Miller et al. 2005, Pawitan et al. 2005, Desmedt et al. 2007a, Minn et al. 2005, Chin et al. 2006) on Affymetrix Human Genome HG-U133A arrays. Survival predictions were fairly concordant across most gene signatures (Zhao et al. Unpublished). We found that these signatures generally performed better in ER positive than in ER negative breast cancers for prediction of distant metastasis free survival (Zhao et al. Unpublished). Cell proliferation seems to be the common driving force for the prognostication in ER positive breast cancers, while different biological mechanisms such as stress response and immune response (Rody et al. 2009, Teschendorff and Caldas 2008) may be crucial for risk stratification in ER negative tumors. The majority of the tested gene signatures are strong risk predictors especially during the first five years of follow-up for distant metastasis free survival and throughout the first 10 years for breast cancer specific survival. These indications are also in line with results from other studies (Desmedt et al. 2007b, Desmedt et al. 2008, Wirapati et al. 2008, Loi et al. 2007). It suggests that different molecular mechanisms are likely to be involved in the early and the late stage during the progression of the metastatic disease.

2.4 Combining multiple gene signatures likely to improve prognosis

Despite the fact that very few genes are shared among various gene signatures, most of gene signatures, evaluated in our own studies (Zhao et al. 2011) and by others (Fan et al. 2006, van Vliet et al. 2008, Reyal et al. 2008), have similar performances in survival risk assessment on the same breast cancer patients. This indicates that some common biological processes overlap across those gene signatures (Reyal et al. 2008, Yu et al. 2007, Desmedt et al. 2008), but more importantly they are likely to capture various biological aspects of breast cancer (Drier and Domany 2011). The combined information from multiple informative gene signatures is arguably more broadly applicable for survival prediction across heterogeneous tumor groups capturing a broad spectrum of biological aspects.

Methods such as decision-tree analysis have been explored to develop a combined predictor that showed improved performance than the individual gene signatures (Chang et al. 2005). In Zhao et al. (Zhao et al. 2011), an analytical framework (Fig. 1) was proposed to improve breast cancer risk stratification by integration of multiple informative gene signatures. We use the gene sets of eleven published gene signatures (Paik et al. 2004, Finak et al. 2008, Minn et al. 2005, van 't Veer et al. 2002, Wang et al. 2005, Sotiriou et al. 2006, van Vliet et al. 2008, Chi et al. 2006, Liu et al. 2007, Hu et al. 2006, Chang et al. 2004) to analyze breast cancer survival and relapse. To investigate the relationship between breast cancer survival and gene expression on a particular gene set, a Cox proportional hazards model is applied using partial likelihood regression with an L2 penalty to avoid overfitting and using cross-validation to determine the penalty weight. The fitted models are applied to an independent test set to obtain a predicted risk index (PI) for each individual and each gene

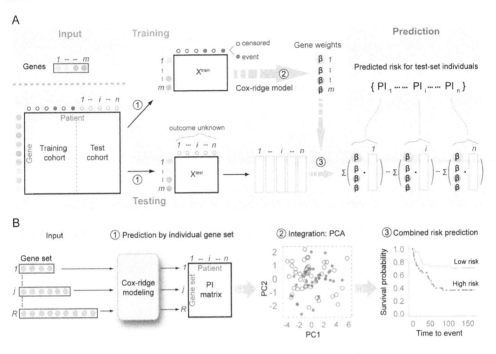

Fig. 1. Flowchart of the analysis showing integration of multiple informative gene signatures.

(A) Construction of the gene-set predictor/gene signature for risk prediction. Input: A set of genes of interest (gene 1, ..., m) which can be traced by the corresponding colors through out the diagram; gene expression data for training cohort and test cohort with genes placed in the rows and patients in the columns. *Step 1.* Gene identity mapping and extract expression matrix. *Step 2.* With available status of observing an event for the patients on the training set, a Cox model with L2 penalty is used to model the relationship of survival probability and gene expression pattern of the gene set. The coefficients or "gene weights" (β_1, ..., β_m) associated with individual genes are estimated from the Cox-ridge model. Size of the bubble in the gene weights matrix reflects the importance of the corresponding gene for survival prediction. *Step 3.* A *Prognostic Index* (PI), the predicted risk score for a test patient i ($i = 1, ..., n$) is calculated by the sum of weighted gene expression from test patient i using the estimated gene weights from step2. (B) Integration of multiple gene signatures by dimension reduction. Input multiple gene sets of interest together with their gene expression data. *Module 1:* For jth gene set ($j = 1, ..., R$), the procedure described in panel A is used to predict a risk score PI for individual test patient. The resulting PI matrix is positioned in R by n dimension representing the risk prediction of the n test patients by each of the R gene sets. *Module 2:* Integrate predictions from multiple gene signatures by dimension reduction using principal components analysis (PCA).

Module 3: Dichotomize the risk scores on PC1 by median (higher than median indicates high risk) resulting in two predicted risk groups for survival outcome. Image is taken from Ref. (Zhao et al. 2011).

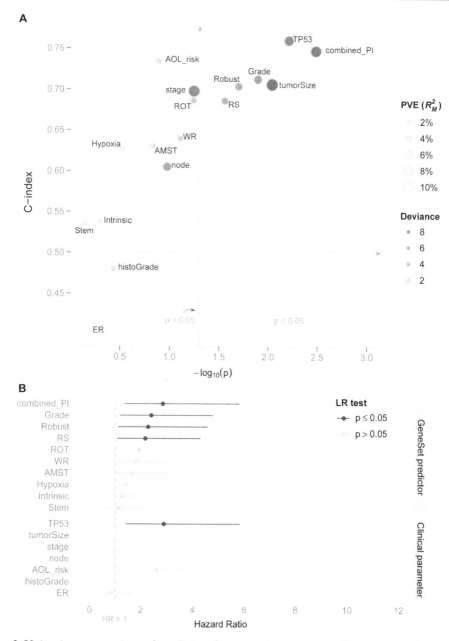

Fig. 2. Univariate comparison of predictors for systemic recurrence. Comparison of combined-PI risk predictor with clinical parameters and individual gene-set predictors using univariate Cox model. **(A)** Y-axis indicates C-index associated with individual predictor and X-axis indicates the p values (on minus log10 scale) from likelihood ratio test in univariate Cox model. C-index = 0.5 and the significant level: $\alpha = 0.05$ for the likelihood

ratio test are indicated by the dotted line. The size and the color of the bubble indicate the PVE and the deviance in univariate Cox model, respectively. The combined-PI risk predictor had the most significant marginal effect for predicting systemic recurrence (p = 0.003). It was associated with the second highest C-index score (C = 0.75) following $TP53$ mutation status (C = 0.76). It had the second highest deviance (8.61) following tumor size (9.36), and the combined-PI predictor alone explained 10.6% of the variability as indicated by PVE, following tumor size (11.7%) and stage (11.1%) **(B)** X-axis indicates HR from the univariate Cox model and the 95% CIs are shown along with the point estimates. "LR test" stands for likelihood ratio test. Insignificant predictors (likelihood ratio test p > 0.05) are grayed out. To keep the results interpretable, only predictors with two levels are compared. The combined-PI risk predictor had the 2nd largest HR (2.82 with 95% CI 1.37−5.80) following $TP53$ mutation status (2.87 with 95% CI 1.42−5.83). Image is taken from Ref. (Zhao et al. 2011).

set. Finally, principal components analysis of the gene signatures is used to derive a combined predictor from the first principal component. Based on a media cut, this combined model classifies test individuals into two risk groups with distinct survival characteristics (recurrence: p=0.003; breast cancer specific death: p=0.001). And it outperforms all the individual gene signatures, as well as Cox models based on traditional clinical parameters and the Adjuvant! Online for survival prediction (Fig. 2).

One weakness of this study is the fact that the training and test sets contain small sample sizes (training set: n = 123; test set: n = 80). The effect of the small sample size is reflected in the low degree of correlation between the PIs obtained by swapping the training and test sets. On the positive side, this study represents an elegant way to combine existing gene sets into a single predictor, without discretizing the survival times. It would be very interesting to see the performance of this classifier on a much larger cohort and explore different approaches for the integration step.

2.5 Clinical trials to conclude the clinical utility of gene expression signatures

To meet the requirements of a prognostic marker, the potential marker should be tested retrospectively in large patient cohorts with a long follow-up period. Subsequently, the findings should be validated by an independent group of experts, and, ideally, a prospective study should confirm the prognostic significance of the tested marker.

Ongoing clinical trials, MINDACT (Microarray In Node negative Disease may Avoid ChemoTherapy) (Cardoso and Van't Veer 2008) and TAILORx (Trial Assigning IndividuaLized Options for Treatment (Rx)) (Sparano and Paik 2008) have been launched to test the clinical usage of MammaPrint® (Agendia, Amsterdam, The Netherlands) (van 't Veer et al. 2002) and Oncotype DX® (Genomic Health Inc., Redwood City, CA) (Paik et al. 2004), respectively. MINDACT will directly compare the 70-gene signature (experimental arm) with Adjuvant! Online (clinico-pathological control arm) to determine whether to offer adjuvant chemotherapy in patients with node-negative breast cancer presenting with discordant risk estimation according to the two methods. It is estimated that 10-15% fewer women will be treated with chemotherapy in the experimental arm. In TAILORx, patients with low RS will be treated with hormonal therapy alone and patients with a high score will receive chemotherapy plus hormonal therapy. However, the 10-year results of both trials will not be available before the year 2020. These trials should provide level I evidence about the clinical relevance of applying gene-expression signatures to daily breast cancer patient management.

In addition, a phase II clinical trial design, the I-SPY 2 (investigation of serial studies to predict your therapeutic response with imaging and molecular analysis 2) (Barker et al. 2009), will test the idea of tailoring treatment by using molecular tests (estrogen receptor status, HER2 status, and the MammaPrint® (Mook et al. 2007, Cardoso and Van't Veer 2008) to identify patients who might benefit from investigational new drugs given along with standard neoadjuvant chemotherapy.

3. Conclusion

Breast cancer is markedly heterogeneous with respect to distinctive biological characteristics and clinical behavior. Many examples highlight that gene expression signatures have tremendous power to identify new cancer subtypes and to predict clinical outcomes. The genome-wide information of breast cancer provides overlapping clinico-pathological classifications, more importantly, adds prognostic accuracy and biological insights than relying on single biomarkers alone.

These signatures are more predictive in ER positive tumors, as seen from our study (Zhao et al. Unpublished) and others. Their low performances in ER negative group are in line with their limitation of assigning the high-risk category to almost all ER-negative patients (Sotiriou and Pusztai 2009, Wirapati et al. 2008). Moreover, their effects on survival prediction seem to decay with time (Desmedt et al. 2007b, Zhao et al. Unpublished), suggesting that different molecular mechanisms are likely involved during the development of early and late stages of the disease.

4. Future of personalized medicine in breast cancer

Genomic signatures play a significant role in individualized diagnosis, prognosis and therapeutic decision-making for cancer patients. In additional to mRNA expression profiling, other genetic information such as genomic complexity inferred from aCGH data (Russnes et al. 2010) also has possibilities to be translated into clinical applications for breast cancer. More recently, next generation DNA sequencing has been used to support the goals of personalized medicine. Charactering complete catalogues of the somatic alterations in cancer genomes holds great potential to discover informative biomarkers and develop targeted therapeutics (Chin et al. 2011).

Clinical and pathological factors such as axillary lymph node status, tumor size, histological grade, histological subtype, HER2 status, and hormone receptor status are still the most important factors for determining treatment. With increasing knowledge of specific genetic alterations and gene expression profiles of tumors, and the prognostic and predictive value of these genetic tumor characteristics, more individualized predictions of disease outcome and refined patient therapy are beginning to be realized.

Integration of clinical, pathological, genetic information derived from gene expression profiling, aCGH and massive parallel sequencing as well as metabolic profiles is a promising approach to achieve better breast cancer risk stratification and further to improve treatment decisions in breast cancer patients. Methods such as PARADIGM (Vaske et al. 2010) have been explored to infer patient-specific signaling pathway activities from integration of multi-dimensional cancer genomics data. Furthermore, the predicted pathway perturbations were able to stratify patients into clinically relevant subtypes (Vaske et al.

2010). With the advances in genomic technologies and the increased volume of high throughput data, it is imperative to develop approaches for integration of diverse biological information – DNA (and epigenetic changes), RNA, proteins and metabolites together with clinical, pathological information.

We look forward to the completion of the ongoing clinical trials to confirm the clinical utility of expression-based gene signatures in breast cancer. We anticipate that these results will facilitate the translation of other genetic information (such as genomic complexity inferred from aCGH data) (Russnes et al. 2010) into clinical applications for breast cancer. We particularly look forward to the impact of next generation DNA sequencing on diagnosis, prognosis and therapeutic decision-making.

5. References

Albain, K. S., W. E. Barlow, S. Shak, G. N. Hortobagyi, R. B. Livingston & I. Yeh (2010) Prognostic and predictive value of the 21-gene recurrence score assay in postmenopausal women with node-positive, oestrogen-receptor-positive breast cancer on chemotherapy: a retrospective analysis of a randomised trial. *The Lancet Oncology*, 11, 55-65.

Bamford, S., E. Dawson, S. Forbes, J. Clements, R. Pettett, A. Dogan, A. Flanagan, J. Teague, P. Futreal & M. Stratton (2004) The COSMIC (Catalogue of Somatic Mutations in Cancer) database and website. *British journal of cancer*, 91, 355-358.

Barker, A., C. Sigman, G. Kelloff, N. Hylton, D. Berry & L. Esserman (2009) I-SPY 2: an adaptive breast cancer trial design in the setting of neoadjuvant chemotherapy. *Clinical Pharmacology & Therapeutics*, 86, 97-100.

Bellman, R. 1961. Adaptive control processes. Princeton University Press, Princeton, NJ.

Bøvelstad, H. M., S. Nygard, H. L. Størvold, M. Aldrin, O. Borgan, A. Frigessi & O. C. Lingjærde (2007) Predicting survival from microarray data--a comparative study. *Bioinformatics*, 23, 2080-7.

Buyse, M., S. Loi, L. Van't Veer, G. Viale, M. Delorenzi, A. M. Glas & A. Saghatchian (2006) Validation and clinical utility of a 70-gene prognostic signature for women with node-negative breast cancer. *JNCI Cancer Spectrum*, 98, 1183.

Cardoso, F. & L. Van't Veer (2008) Clinical application of the 70-gene profile: the MINDACT trial. *Journal of Clinical Oncology*, 26, 729.

Carter, C. L., C. Allen & D. E. Henson (1989) Relation of tumor size, lymph node status, and survival in 24,740 breast cancer cases. *Cancer*, 63, 181-187.

Chang, H. Y., D. S. A. Nuyten, J. B. Sneddon, T. Hastie, R. Tibshirani, T. Sørlie, H. Dai, Y. D. He, L. J. Van't Veer & H. Bartelink (2005) Robustness, scalability, and integration of a wound-response gene expression signature in predicting breast cancer survival. *Proceedings of the National Academy of Sciences of the United States of America*, 102, 3738.

Chang, H. Y., J. B. Sneddon, A. A. Alizadeh, R. Sood, R. B. West, K. Montgomery, J. T. Chi, M. van de Rijn, D. Botstein & P. O. Brown (2004) Gene expression signature of fibroblast serum response predicts human cancer progression: similarities between tumors and wounds. *PLoS Biol*, 2, E7.

Chi, J. T., Z. Wang, D. S. Nuyten, E. H. Rodriguez, M. E. Schaner, A. Salim, Y. Wang, G. B. Kristensen, A. Helland, A. L. Borresen-Dale, A. Giaccia, M. T. Longaker, T. Hastie, G. P. Yang, M. J. van de Vijver & P. O. Brown (2006) Gene expression programs in response to hypoxia: cell type specificity and prognostic significance in human cancers. *PLoS Med*, 3, e47.

Chin, K., S. DeVries, J. Fridlyand, P. T. Spellman, R. Roydasgupta, W. L. Kuo, A. Lapuk, R. M. Neve, Z. Qian & T. Ryder (2006) Genomic and transcriptional aberrations linked to breast cancer pathophysiologies. *Cancer Cell*, 10, 529-541.

Chin, L., J. N. Andersen & P. A. Futreal (2011) Cancer genomics: from discovery science to personalized medicine. *Nature medicine*, 17, 297-303.

Chustecka, Z. (2007) Survival Disadvantage Seen for Triple-Negative Breast Cancer.

Cohen, J. (1960) A coefficient of agreement for nominal scales. *Educational and psychological measurement*, 20, 37-46.

Dent, R., M. Trudeau, K. I. Pritchard, W. M. Hanna, H. K. Kahn, C. A. Sawka, L. A. Lickley, E. Rawlinson, P. Sun & S. A. Narod (2007) Triple-negative breast cancer: clinical features and patterns of recurrence. *Clinical Cancer Research*, 13, 4429.

Desmedt, C., B. Haibe-Kains, P. Wirapati, M. Buyse, D. Larsimont, G. Bontempi, M. Delorenzi, M. Piccart & C. Sotiriou (2008) Biological processes associated with breast cancer clinical outcome depend on the molecular subtypes. *Clinical Cancer Research*, 14, 5158.

Desmedt, C., F. Piette, S. Loi, Y. Wang, F. Lallemand, B. Haibe-Kains, G. Viale, M. Delorenzi, Y. Zhang & M. d'Assignies (2007a) TRANSBIG Consortium. Strong time dependence of the 76-gene prognostic signature for node-negative breast cancer patients in the TRANSBIG multicenter independent validation series. *Clin Cancer Res*, 13, 3207-14.

Desmedt, C., F. Piette, S. Loi, Y. Wang, F. Lallemand, B. Haibe-Kains, G. Viale, M. Delorenzi, Y. Zhang & M. S. d'Assignies (2007b) Strong time dependence of the 76-gene prognostic signature for node-negative breast cancer patients in the TRANSBIG multicenter independent validation series. *Clinical Cancer Research*, 13, 3207.

Drier, Y. & E. Domany (2011) Do Two Machine-Learning Based Prognostic Signatures for Breast Cancer Capture the Same Biological Processes? *PLoS One*, 6, e17795.

Espinosa, E., J. Vara, A. Redondo, J. Sanchez, D. Hardisson, P. Zamora, F. G. Pastrana, P. Cejas, B. Martinez & A. Suarez (2005) Breast cancer prognosis determined by gene expression profiling: a quantitative reverse transcriptase polymerase chain reaction study. *Journal of Clinical Oncology*, 23, 7278.

Fan, C., D. S. Oh, L. Wessels, B. Weigelt, D. S. Nuyten, A. B. Nobel, L. J. van't Veer & C. M. Perou (2006) Concordance among gene-expression-based predictors for breast cancer. *N Engl J Med*, 355, 560-9.

Finak, G., N. Bertos, F. Pepin, S. Sadekova, M. Souleimanova, H. Zhao, H. Chen, G. Omeroglu, S. Meterissian, A. Omeroglu, M. Hallett & M. Park (2008) Stromal gene expression predicts clinical outcome in breast cancer. *Nat Med*, 14, 518-27.

Fisher, B., C. Redmond, E. R. Fisher & R. Caplan (1988) Relative worth of estrogen or progesterone receptor and pathologic characteristics of differentiation as indicators of prognosis in node negative breast cancer patients: findings from National Surgical Adjuvant Breast and Bowel Project Protocol B-06. *Journal of Clinical Oncology*, 6, 1076.

Foekens, J. A., D. Atkins, Y. Zhang, F. C. G. J. Sweep, N. Harbeck, A. Paradiso, T. Cufer, A. M. Sieuwerts, D. Talantov & P. N. Span (2006) Multicenter validation of a gene expressionñbased prognostic signature in lymph nodeñnegative primary breast cancer. *Journal of Clinical Oncology*, 24, 1665.

Frank, I. & J. Friedman (1993) A statistical view of some chemometrics regression tools. *Technometrics*, 35, 109-135.

Garcia, M., A. Jemal, E. Ward, M. Center, Y. Hao, R. Siegel & M. Thun (2007) Global cancer facts & figures 2007. *Atlanta, GA: American Cancer Society*, 1.

Haibe-Kains, B., C. Desmedt, F. Piette, M. Buyse, F. Cardoso, L. Van't Veer, M. Piccart, G. Bontempi & C. Sotiriou (2008a) Comparison of prognostic gene expression signatures for breast cancer. *BMC Genomics, 9*, 394.

Haibe-Kains, B., C. Desmedt, C. Sotiriou & G. Bontempi (2008b) A comparative study of survival models for breast cancer prognostication based on microarray data: does a single gene beat them all? *Bioinformatics, 24*, 2200.

Hastie, T., R. Tibshirani & J. Friedman (2001) The elements of statistical learning: data mining, inference, and prediction. *New York: Springer-Verlag, 1*, 371-406.

Haybittle, J., R. Blamey, C. Elston, J. Johnson, P. Doyle, F. Campbell, R. Nicholson & K. Griffiths (1982) A prognostic index in primary breast cancer. *British journal of cancer, 45*, 361.

Hu, Z., C. Fan, D. S. Oh, J. S. Marron, X. He, B. F. Qaqish, C. Livasy, L. A. Carey, E. Reynolds, L. Dressler, A. Nobel, J. Parker, M. G. Ewend, L. R. Sawyer, J. Wu, Y. Liu, R. Nanda, M. Tretiakova, A. Ruiz Orrico, D. Dreher, J. P. Palazzo, L. Perreard, E. Nelson, M. Mone, H. Hansen, M. Mullins, J. F. Quackenbush, M. J. Ellis, O. I. Olopade, P. S. Bernard & C. M. Perou (2006) The molecular portraits of breast tumors are conserved across microarray platforms. *BMC Genomics, 7*, 96.

Koscielny, S., M. Tubiana, M. Le, A. Valleron, H. Mouriesse, G. Contesso & D. Sarrazin (1984) Breast cancer: relationship between the size of the primary tumour and the probability of metastatic dissemination. *British journal of cancer, 49*, 709.

Lingjærde, O. C. & N. Christophersen (2000) Shrinkage structure of partial least squares. *Scandinavian Journal of Statistics, 27*, 459-473.

Liu, R., X. Wang, G. Y. Chen, P. Dalerba, A. Gurney, T. Hoey, G. Sherlock, J. Lewicki, K. Shedden & M. F. Clarke (2007) The prognostic role of a gene signature from tumorigenic breast-cancer cells. *N Engl J Med, 356*, 217-26.

Loi, S., B. Haibe-Kains, C. Desmedt, F. Lallemand, A. M. Tutt, C. Gillet, P. Ellis, A. Harris, J. Bergh & J. A. Foekens (2007) Definition of clinically distinct molecular subtypes in estrogen receptor-positive breast carcinomas through genomic grade. *Journal of Clinical Oncology, 25*, 1239.

Miller, L. D., J. Smeds, J. George, V. B. Vega, L. Vergara, A. Ploner, Y. Pawitan, P. Hall, S. Klaar & E. T. Liu (2005) An expression signature for p53 status in human breast cancer predicts mutation status, transcriptional effects, and patient survival. *Proceedings of the National Academy of Sciences of the United States of America, 102*, 13550.

Minn, A. J., G. P. Gupta, P. M. Siegel, P. D. Bos, W. Shu, D. D. Giri, A. Viale, A. B. Olshen, W. L. Gerald & J. Massague (2005) Genes that mediate breast cancer metastasis to lung. *Nature, 436*, 518-24.

Mook, S., M. K. Schmidt, G. Viale, G. Pruneri, I. Eekhout, A. Floore, A. M. Glas, J. Bogaerts, F. Cardoso, M. J. Piccart-Gebhart, E. T. Rutgers, L. J. Van't Veer & T. c. On behalf of the (2008) The 70-gene prognosis-signature predicts disease outcome in breast cancer patients with 1-3 positive lymph nodes in an independent validation study. *Breast Cancer Res Treat.*

Mook, S., L. J. Van't Veer, E. J. Rutgers, M. J. Piccart-Gebhart & F. Cardoso (2007) Individualization of therapy using Mammaprint: from development to the MINDACT Trial. *Cancer genomics & proteomics, 4*, 147.

Nuyten, D. S. A., T. Hastie, J. T. A. Chi, H. Y. Chang & M. J. van de Vijver (2008) Combining biological gene expression signatures in predicting outcome in breast cancer: An alternative to supervised classification. *European Journal of Cancer, 44*, 2319-2329.

Page, D. L. (1991) Prognosis and breast cancer: recognition of lethal and favorable prognostic types. *The American Journal of Surgical Pathology,* 15, 334.

Paik, S., S. Shak, G. Tang, C. Kim, J. Baker, M. Cronin, F. L. Baehner, M. G. Walker, D. Watson, T. Park, W. Hiller, E. R. Fisher, D. L. Wickerham, J. Bryant & N. Wolmark (2004) A multigene assay to predict recurrence of tamoxifen-treated, node-negative breast cancer. *N Engl J Med,* 351, 2817-26.

Parker, J. S., M. Mullins, M. C. U. Cheang, S. Leung, D. Voduc, T. Vickery, S. Davies, C. Fauron, X. He & Z. Hu (2009) Supervised risk predictor of breast cancer based on intrinsic subtypes. *Journal of Clinical Oncology,* 27, 1160.

Pawitan, Y., J. Bjöhle, L. Amler, A. L. Borg, S. Egyhazi, P. Hall, X. Han, L. Holmberg, F. Huang & S. Klaar (2005) Gene expression profiling spares early breast cancer patients from adjuvant therapy: derived and validated in two population-based cohorts. *Breast Cancer Research,* 7, R953-R964.

Perou, C. M., S. S. Jeffrey, M. van de Rijn, C. A. Rees, M. B. Eisen, D. T. Ross, A. Pergamenschikov, C. F. Williams, S. X. Zhu, J. C. F. Lee, D. Lashkari, D. Shalon, P. O. Brown & D. Botstein (1999) Distinctive gene expression patterns in human mammary epithelial cells and breast cancers. *Proceedings of the National Academy of Sciences,* 96, 9212-9217.

Perou, C. M., T. Sørlie, M. B. Eisen, M. van de Rijn, S. S. Jeffrey, C. A. Rees, J. R. Pollack, D. T. Ross, H. Johnsen, L. A. Akslen, O. Fluge, A. Pergamenschikov, C. Williams, S. X. Zhu, P. E. Lonning, A. L. Børresen-Dale, P. O. Brown & D. Botstein (2000) Molecular portraits of human breast tumours. *Nature,* 406, 747-52.

Perreard, L., C. Fan, J. F. Quackenbush, M. Mullins, N. P. Gauthier, E. Nelson, M. Mone, H. Hansen, S. S. Buys & K. Rasmussen (2006) Classification and risk stratification of invasive breast carcinomas using a real-time quantitative RT-PCR assay. *Breast Cancer Res,* 8, R23.

Prat, A. & C. M. Perou (2009) Mammary development meets cancer genomics. *Nature medicine,* 15, 842-844.

Ravdin, P., L. Siminoff, G. Davis, M. Mercer, J. Hewlett, N. Gerson & H. Parker (2001) Computer program to assist in making decisions about adjuvant therapy for women with early breast cancer. *Journal of Clinical Oncology,* 19, 980.

Reyal, F., M. Van Vliet, N. Armstrong, H. Horlings, K. De Visser, M. Kok, A. Teschendorff, S. Mook, L. Van't Veer & C. Caldas (2008) A comprehensive analysis of prognostic signatures reveals the high predictive capacity of the proliferation, immune response and RNA splicing modules in breast cancer. *Breast Cancer Res,* 10, R93.

Rody, A., U. Holtrich, L. Pusztai, C. Liedtke, R. Gaetje, E. Ruckhaeberle, C. Solbach, L. Hanker, A. Ahr, D. Metzler, K. Engels, T. Karn & M. Kaufmann (2009) T-cell metagene predicts a favorable prognosis in estrogen receptor-negative and HER2-positive breast cancers. *Breast Cancer Res,* 11, R15.

Rønneberg, J. A., T. Fleischer, H. K. Solvang, S. H. Nordgard, H. Edvardsen, I. Potapenko, D. Nebdal, C. Daviaud, I. Gut, I. Bukholm, N. B., B.-D. A.L., T. J. & K. V. (2010) Methylation profiling with a panel of cancer related genes: Association with estrogen receptor, TP53 mutation status and expression subtypes in sporadic breast cancer. *Molecular Oncology.*

Rosen, P. P., S. Groshen, P. E. Saigo, D. W. Kinne & S. Hellman (1989) Pathological prognostic factors in stage I (T1N0M0) and stage II (T1N1M0) breast carcinoma: a study of 644 patients with median follow-up of 18 years. *Journal of Clinical Oncology,* 7, 1239.

Rousseeuw, P. J. (1987) Silhouettes: a graphical aid to the interpretation and validation of cluster analysis. *Journal of computational and applied mathematics*, 20, 53-65.

Russnes, H., H. Vollan, O. Lingjærde, A. Krasnitz, P. Lundin, B. Naume, T. Sørlie, E. Borgen, I. Rye & A. Langerød (2010) Genomic Architecture Characterizes Tumor Progression Paths and Fate in Breast Cancer Patients. *Science Translational Medicine*, 2, 38ra47.

Scarff, R. W., H. Torloni & W. H. Organization. 1968. *Histological typing of breast tumours*. World Health Organization.

Slamon, D. J., W. Godolphin, L. A. Jones, J. A. Holt, S. G. Wong, D. E. Keith, W. J. Levin, S. G. Stuart, J. Udove & A. Ullrich (1989) Studies of the HER-2/neu proto-oncogene in human breast and ovarian cancer. *Science*, 244, 707.

Smyth, G. K. (2004) Linear models and empirical Bayes methods for assessing differential expression in microarray experiments. *Statistical applications in genetics and molecular biology*, 3, 3.

Smyth, G. K., J. Michaud & H. S. Scott (2005) Use of within-array replicate spots for assessing differential expression in microarray experiments. *Bioinformatics*, 21, 2067.

Sørlie, T., E. Borgan, S. Myhre, H. K. Vollan, H. Russnes, X. Zhao, G. Nilsen, O. C. Lingjærde, A. L. Børresen-Dale & E. Rødland (2010) The importance of gene-centring microarray data. *The Lancet Oncology*, 11, 719-720.

Sørlie, T., C. M. Perou, R. Tibshirani, T. Aas, S. Geisler, H. Johnsen, T. Hastie, M. B. Eisen, M. van de Rijn, S. S. Jeffrey, T. Thorsen, H. Quist, J. C. Matese, P. O. Brown, D. Botstein, P. Eystein Lonning & A. L. Børresen-Dale (2001) Gene expression patterns of breast carcinomas distinguish tumor subclasses with clinical implications. *Proc Natl Acad Sci U S A*, 98, 10869-74.

Sørlie, T., R. Tibshirani, J. Parker, T. Hastie, J. S. Marron, A. Nobel, S. Deng, H. Johnsen, R. Pesich, S. Geisler, J. Demeter, C. M. Perou, P. E. Lonning, P. O. Brown, A. L. Borresen-Dale & D. Botstein (2003) Repeated observation of breast tumor subtypes in independent gene expression data sets. *Proc Natl Acad Sci U S A*, 100, 8418-23.

Sotiriou, C. & L. Pusztai (2009) Gene-expression signatures in breast cancer. *New England Journal of Medicine*, 360, 790-800.

Sotiriou, C., P. Wirapati, S. Loi, A. Harris, S. Fox, J. Smeds, H. Nordgren, P. Farmer, V. Praz, B. Haibe-Kains, C. Desmedt, D. Larsimont, F. Cardoso, H. Peterse, D. Nuyten, M. Buyse, M. J. Van de Vijver, J. Bergh, M. Piccart & M. Delorenzi (2006) Gene expression profiling in breast cancer: understanding the molecular basis of histologic grade to improve prognosis. *J Natl Cancer Inst*, 98, 262-72.

Sparano, J. A. & S. Paik (2008) Development of the 21-gene assay and its application in clinical practice and clinical trials. *Journal of Clinical Oncology*, 26, 721.

Stephens, P. J., D. J. McBride, M. L. Lin, I. Varela, E. D. Pleasance, J. T. Simpson, L. A. Stebbings, C. Leroy, S. Edkins & L. J. Mudie (2009) Complex landscapes of somatic rearrangement in human breast cancer genomes. *Nature*, 462, 1005-1010.

Suzuki, R. & H. Shimodaira. 2004. An application of multiscale bootstrap resampling to hierarchical clustering of microarray data: How accurate are these clusters. 34.

Teschendorff, A. E. & C. Caldas (2008) A robust classifier of high predictive value to identify good prognosis patients in ER-negative breast cancer. *Breast Cancer Res*, 10, R73.

Tibshirani, R. (1996) Regression shrinkage and selection via the lasso. *Journal of the Royal Statistical Society. Series B (Methodological)*, 267-288.

Tibshirani, R., G. Walther & T. Hastie (2001) Estimating the number of clusters in a data set via the gap statistic. *Journal of the Royal Statistical Society: Series B (Statistical Methodology)*, 63, 411-423.

Tusher, V. G., R. Tibshirani & G. Chu (2001) Significance analysis of microarrays applied to the ionizing radiation response. *Proceedings of the National Academy of Sciences of the United States of America*, 98, 5116.

van 't Veer, L. J., H. Dai, M. J. van de Vijver, Y. D. He, A. A. Hart, M. Mao, H. L. Peterse, K. van der Kooy, M. J. Marton, A. T. Witteveen, G. J. Schreiber, R. M. Kerkhoven, C. Roberts, P. S. Linsley, R. Bernards & S. H. Friend (2002) Gene expression profiling predicts clinical outcome of breast cancer. *Nature*, 415, 530-6.

van de Vijver, M. J., Y. D. He, L. J. van't Veer, H. Dai, A. A. Hart, D. W. Voskuil, G. J. Schreiber, J. L. Peterse, C. Roberts, M. J. Marton, M. Parrish, D. Atsma, A. Witteveen, A. Glas, L. Delahaye, T. van der Velde, H. Bartelink, S. Rodenhuis, E. T. Rutgers, S. H. Friend & R. Bernards (2002) A gene-expression signature as a predictor of survival in breast cancer. *N Engl J Med*, 347, 1999-2009.

van Vliet, M. H., F. Reyal, H. M. Horlings, M. J. van de Vijver, M. J. Reinders & L. F. Wessels (2008) Pooling breast cancer datasets has a synergetic effect on classification performance and improves signature stability. *BMC Genomics*, 9, 375.

Vaske, C. J., S. C. Benz, J. Z. Sanborn, D. Earl, C. Szeto, J. Zhu, D. Haussler & J. M. Stuart (2010) Inference of patient-specific pathway activities from multi-dimensional cancer genomics data using PARADIGM. *Bioinformatics*, 26, i237.

Verweij, P. J. & H. C. Van Houwelingen (1993) Cross-validation in survival analysis. *Stat Med*, 12, 2305-14.

Verweij, P. J. & H. C. Van Houwelingen (1994) Penalized likelihood in Cox regression. *Stat Med*, 13, 2427-36.

Wang, Y., J. G. Klijn, Y. Zhang, A. M. Sieuwerts, M. P. Look, F. Yang, D. Talantov, M. Timmermans, M. E. Meijer-van Gelder, J. Yu, T. Jatkoe, E. M. Berns, D. Atkins & J. A. Foekens (2005) Gene-expression profiles to predict distant metastasis of lymph-node-negative primary breast cancer. *Lancet*, 365, 671-9.

Weigelt, B., J. L. Peterse & L. J. van't Veer (2005) Breast cancer metastasis: markers and models. *Nature Reviews Cancer*, 5, 591-602.

Wirapati, P., C. Sotiriou, S. Kunkel, P. Farmer, S. Pradervand, B. Haibe-Kains, C. Desmedt, M. Ignatiadis, T. Sengstag & F. Schutz (2008) Meta-analysis of gene expression profiles in breast cancer: toward a unified understanding of breast cancer subtyping and prognosis signatures. *Breast Cancer Res*, 10, R65.

Yu, J. X., A. M. Sieuwerts, Y. Zhang, J. W. Martens, M. Smid, J. G. Klijn, Y. Wang & J. A. Foekens (2007) Pathway analysis of gene signatures predicting metastasis of node-negative primary breast cancer. *BMC Cancer*, 7, 182.

Zhao, X., E. A. Rødland, T. Sørlie, B. Naume, A. Langerød, A. Frigessi, V. N. Kristensen, A. L. Børresen-Dale & O. C. Lingjærde (2011) Combining Gene Signatures Improves Prediction of Breast Cancer Survival. *PLoS One*, 6, e17845.

Zhao, X., E. A. Rødland, T. Sørlie, H. K. M. Vollan, V. N. Kristensen, O. C. Lingjærde & A. L. Børresen-Dale (Unpublished) Systematic assessment of prognostic gene signatures for breast cancer shows distinct influence of time and ER status.

Zou, H. & T. Hastie (2005) Regularization and variable selection via the elastic net. *Journal of the Royal Statistical Society: Series B (Statistical Methodology)*, 67, 301-320.

8

New Models for
the *In Vitro* Study of Liver Toxicity:
3D Culture Systems and the Role of Bioreactors

Giovanna Mazzoleni and Nathalie Steimberg
Laboratory of Tissue Engineering, General Pathology & Immunology Unit
Faculty of Medicine and Surgery, University of Brescia,
Italy

1. Introduction

Present in all animal species, even if less developed in the lowest classes of the animal kingdom, the liver fulfils many vital functions of the utmost importance for the organism's survival. In adult humans, the biological significance of liver is attested by its anatomical localisation, its volume, its complexity, and by the density of the cellular elements it is composed of. Located in the right upper quadrant of the abdominal cavity, just below the diaphragm (Fig. 1), the liver represents, as a matter of fact, the largest visceral organ in the human body (about 2.5% of the dry body weight of an adult), and its parenchyma is constituted of more than 300 billion cells (Conti, 2005).

Physiological investigations have assigned to the liver a complex array of more than 500 different functions, the majority of which still remain unknown in their molecular mechanisms and controls. These functions include a number of key metabolic and regulatory activities, as well as processes crucial to the organism's defence (Arias *et al.*, 2009). The principal hepatic functions are schematised in Fig. 2. Indeed, besides carrying a central role in the metabolism of carbohydrates, lipids and proteins, the liver regulates other critical homeostatic functions, such as endocrine activity and haemostasis (synthesis/activation/catabolism of hormonal compounds, and of the majority of coagulation's/fibrinolysis' factors and inhibitors), and it directly acts as an integrant part of the systemic reaction to injury by, for example, modulating the immune response and synthesizing proteins from the "acute phase" (Nahmias *et al.*, 2006). In addition to its multiple metabolic activities, the liver also represents the first line of defence of the whole organism against exogenous or toxic substances. The liver is, in effect, the major site for inactivation of toxins and xenobiotics, favours their removal from the blood and further elimination from the organism through bile secretion (processes of biotransformation and excretion) [1] (Arias *et al.*, 2009).

---

[1] **Biotransformation of drugs, xenobiotics, toxins and endogenous compounds.**
Part of lipophilic compounds can accumulate in the body (mainly in fat and bone tissues) or, alternatively, they need to be transformed in hydrophilic substances, in order to be more readily eliminated (excreted). Most of drugs are poorly hydrosoluble, and are metabolised (biotransformed) mainly at the hepatic level. Biotransformation process is the principal factor that can affect the overall

The importance of this organ and the impossibility to substitute artificially its multiple activities, justify, therefore, the serious clinical consequences of its dysfunction: until now, in industrialized countries, liver failure (acute and chronic) is among the top ten most frequent causes of death (Popovic & Kozak, 1998). A fundamental and typical feature of liver lies in the species-specificity of its functional characteristics and susceptibility to injury, elements that, both, make animal models commonly used for patho-physiological and pharmaco-toxicological studies, inadequate and poorly informative (or predictive) for humans (Rangarajan *et al.*, 2004; Sivaraman *et al.*, 2005). Examples are adverse drug reactions that occur in humans, which, being specifically based on liver metabolism or on hepatocellular sensitivity, are unpredictable or poorly understood (Park *et al.*, 2005).

To date, notwithstanding the long time period required (more than ten years), and the high financial investment necessary for the development of any new drug (estimated at around one billion Euros per molecule, of which, at least, one-fifth is used exclusively for toxicological investigations on hepatic function), almost two-thirds of the compounds that reach the phase III of clinical trials, demonstrate significant hepatotoxic effects in humans, which prevent their approval. Moreover, it is noteworthy that the hepatic toxicity (including idiosyncratic and chronic toxicity) unpredicted by the current experimental protocols represents more than one third of all the causes responsible for the withdrawal from the market of already approved drugs (O'Brien *et al.*, 2004; Whitebread *et al.*, 2005). Lastly, drug-induced hepatotoxicity is a major clinical pitfall, accounting for 50% of all cases of acute liver failure. From the above considerations, it is, therefore, clear how liver plays a unique and central role in toxicological studies: first, because it is critical in the pharmacokinetics of chemicals, due to its functions of biotransformation and excretion of substances, and, second, since it represent a foremost target of organ-specific adverse effects of drugs and xenobiotics.

In order to lessen and offset hepatotoxic effects, a large number of methods were developed and are currently applied in risk assessment procedures (*in vitro* and *in vivo* methods, human clinical trials, clinical case reports, etc.), or in toxicological/epidemiological studies (observation of the exposure-induced effects on human health), aimed to identify potential human hazards. Some of these methods are presented in Table 1, focusing on their features in relation to the fundamental characteristics required to fulfil the process of risk assessment.

---

therapeutic and toxic profile of a drug; it can lead to detoxification, excretion, or, less frequently, to bioactivation of the chemical compound, being, thus, responsible for its biological activity, pharmacokinetics and clearance (Brandon *et al.*, 2003). Biotransformation occurs in three different phases: metabolic phases I and II, and transport phase III. The phase I reactions (functionalization step) include oxidation, reduction, or hydrolysis enzymatic reactions, that are, mainly, catalysed by the cytochrome P450 (CYP)-depending and flavin monooxygenase superfamily enzymes. Part of these phase I metabolites can be eliminated by biliary excretion, whereas another part can be metabolised by the phase II reactions, which allow to conjugate polar compounds (and metabolites) to water-soluble groups (glucuronic acid, sulphate, acetate, glycine, glutathione or methyl and acetyl groups), that render the derivatives much more soluble. Hydrophilic derivatives can then be excreted (mainly by kidney, even if liver excretion through bile also takes place). The third phase of compound biotransformation involves active membrane transporters, which, in hepatocytes, are located at their two polar surface domains. Apical and canalicular ATP-binding cassette (ABC) family of drug transporters are responsible for xenobiotic clearance (or bile secretion); basolateral solute carrier transporters, such as, for example, organic anion transporters (OATs), organic cation transporters (OCTs), and organic anion-transporting polypeptides (OATPs), are involved in the uptake of compound from the blood (Pauli-Magnus & Meier, 2003; Omiecinski *et al.*, 2010).

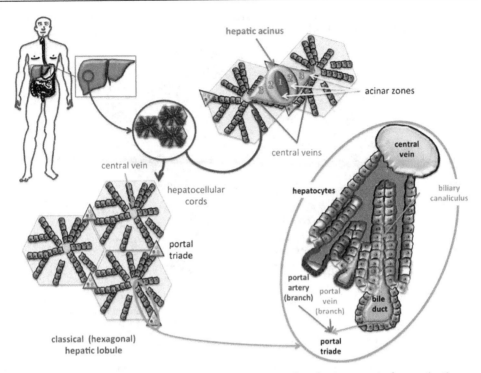

Fig. 1. Schematic view of the liver: location, macroscopical and microscopical organisation.

Since each model possesses advantages (and limits), the most promising strategy to assess the toxicological risk of substances and drugs, should be, at present, a combination of all the information obtained from these various models (integrated testing strategy). Table 2 lists the principal models currently used for hepatotoxicity studies.

Nevertheless, the predictive value for humans of current pre-clinical safety assessment systems is still limited and largely insufficient for a correct estimation of clinically relevant drug-drug interactions (DDIs) and pharmacodynamics/toxicological properties of compounds (ADMET profile) (Soars et al., 2007). Significant inter-individual variability and great inter-species differences in liver functions, that make animal models inadequate for the safety testing of drugs and xenobiotics, have produced the necessity to develop new *in vitro* models, able to better reproduce or mimic the function of the human liver. In the last decades this necessity has already stimulated intense research activity, sustained by significant financial investments. The development of methods (and models) alternative to animal experimentation, along with the approval of their use, either in basic research, or in the more complex field of pharmaco-toxicology, has known a noteworthy expansion in the last twenty years[2] (see Table 2).

---

[2] **"Alternative" methods and the 3R's principle.**
In 1959, Russel and Burch introduced, for the first time, the concept of methods "alternative" to experimental animal models (Russel & Burch, 1959). The authors defined as "alternative" any method that can be used in order to *Replace, Reduce* and *Refine* (3R's principle) the use of animals in biomedical

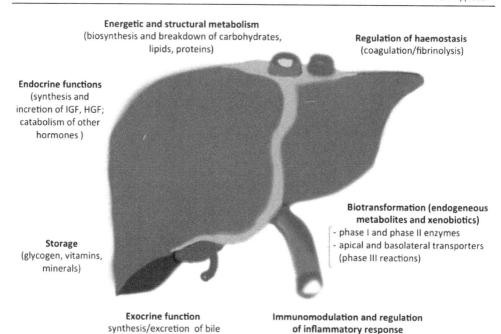

Energetic and structural metabolism
(biosynthesis and breakdown of carbohydrates,
lipids, proteins)

Regulation of haemostasis
(coagulation/fibrinolysis)

Endocrine functions
(synthesis and
incretion of IGF, HGF;
catabolism of other
hormones)

Biotransformation (endogeneous
metabolites and xenobiotics)
- phase I and phase II enzymes
- apical and basolateral transporters
(phase III reactions)

Storage
(glycogen, vitamins,
minerals)

Exocrine function
synthesis/excretion of bile

Immunomodulation and regulation
of inflammatory response

Fig. 2. Schematic representation of the principal liver's functions.

However, due to the high level of specialisation and complexity of the hepatic parenchyma, with its specific intra-lobular "zonal" organisation (Christoffles *et al.*, 1999), and given the peculiar sensibility of its cellular elements to even minimal environmental changes, none among the traditional and more widespread *in vitro* liver-derived models routinely available, seems to possess satisfactory features to be considered as a suitable model of the organ *in vivo* (Brandon *et al.*, 2003; Guillouzo & Guguen-Guillouzo, 2008). New approaches require, actually, the generation (and validation) of human-specific *in vitro* liver-derived test

research, testing or education. The basis of the 3R's principle is the aim to improve ethical standards and animal welfare in *in vivo* experimental procedures, by: i) **replacing**, as much as possible, *in vivo* models (use of alternative methods, i.e. *in vitro*, *ex vivo* and *in silico* approaches), ii) **reducing** the number of animals needed for experimental objectives, and iii) **refining** the experimental procedures, in order to reduce animal sufferance (pain, stress, discomfort). Until now, despite the great political and economical efforts that have been undertaken worldwide during the last two decades (especially by EU, US and other industrialised countries, such as Canada and Japan) to comply with the 3R's strategy (Mazzoleni and Steimberg, 2010; Hartung, 2010), only few alternative methods have been validated for regulatory toxicology and efficacy testing of chemicals. The Organization for Economic Co-Operation and Development (OECD), which represents 30 countries in the Americas (including the United States), Europe, and Asia, provides a collection of internationally harmonized testing methods for a number of toxicological endpoints using *in vivo*, *in vitro*, and even alternative approaches (OECD "Guidelines for the Testing of Chemicals"). For up-to-date information on the *Alternatives to Animal Testing*, see also "**Altweb** - the Alternatives to Animal Testing Web Site" http://altweb.jhsph.edu/), and, for specific bibliography, "**ALTBIB** - Resources on Alternatives to the Use of Live Vertebrates in Biomedical Research and Testing" at http://toxnet.nlm.nih.gov/altbib.html. On the web, **AltTox.org**, is a website dedicated to advancing non-animal methods of toxicity testing through online discussion and information exchange (http://alttox.org/).

Method → / Remark ↓		*In vitro* (cell-based studies)	*In vivo* (animal-based studies)	Human clinical trials (volunteers)	Evidence-based toxicology, human exposure, epidemiology
Reliability of the predictive studies	single organ/tissue	+/-	+/-	++	+++
	whole human population: multifactorial aspects, sex, race age, healthy or pathological conditions	-	-	+/-	+++
Capability to mirror whole organism's response (systemic response, immune and hormonal regulation; all aspects of ADMET and DIDs) (*)		--	+++	+++	+++
Specific toxicity assessment (targeting liver-specific effects and "zonal" toxicity) (**)		-/+	++	++	++++
Range of lethal and non lethal endpoints (acute toxicity)		+++ (IC50)	++ (DL50 + LOEL)	--	Not applicable
Chronic toxicity assessment		-	++	+/-	+++
Wide-range investigations (time-/dose-dependent studies without inter-individual variability, repeated-dose effects, etc.)		+++	++	-	+++
Complex mixtures testing		+++	+++	-	+
Mechanistic studies		+++	++	+/-	+/- (macroscopic effect)
Reproducibility (control of experimental/testing conditions)		+++	+/-	+/-	-
Validation of the systems		+ (some endpoints)	++	Not applicable	Not applicable

Method ➤ ------------ Remark ⬇	In vitro (cell-based studies)	In vivo (animal-based studies)	Human clinical trials (volunteers)	Evidence-based toxicology, human exposure, epidemiology
Ethical features (3R's principle; environmental reduction of potentially toxic wastes, etc.)	+++	-	+	+++
Cost	+	++++	++++	++
General remarks	Validated models are still insufficient to be fully predictive for humans	Animal use, even if still necessary, should be reduced as much as possible	Should be performed after exhaustive pre-clinical studies on accurate/ validated models	By reducing pre-clinical, clinical and post-clinical toxicity, epidemiological studies could be reduced

(*) ADMET: absorption, distribution, metabolism, excretion, and toxicity; DIDs: drug-drug interactions.
(**) Zonal toxicity: specific peri-central/peri-portal toxic effects (Allen *et al.*, 2005).

Table 1. Comparison of the various liver models employed in hepatotoxicity studies.

model systems, which are able to give answers at the physiological level, and to be relevant to human outcomes. While consistent evidence demonstrates the breaking points of traditional *in vitro* models (static culture in monolayer) in reproducing the behaviour and physiological response of various tissues (the hepatic one, in particular), contemporarily, three-dimensional (3D) systems are achieving an increasing status (Mazzoleni *et al.*, 2009). In effect, the more promising results seem, at present, to derive from the 3D techniques of culture, that, by guaranteeing the preservation of at least some characteristics of the complex hepatic microenvironment, can favour cell survival and the *in vitro* expression of the liver-specific differentiated phenotype, allowing, in such a way, the generation of more reliable and predictive hepatic test models for human investigations (Shvartsman *et al.*, 2009).

In the present chapter, the principal models available for the *in vitro* study of liver functions are reviewed. Moreover, the contribution of new emerging technologies and tissue engineering, as basis for the conception of innovative hepatic models, the relevance of 3D bio-constructs, as reliable liver analogues, and their relative advantages and drawbacks in the process of being developed/validated, is discussed. A particular attention is given to the model systems based on the use of dynamic bioreactors, and, more specifically, on the use of the *Rotary Cell Culture System* (RCCS™, Synthecon, Inc.) device.

2. Currently available liver-derived *in vitro* models and the role of liver-specific microenvironment

The need for studying hepatic functions, and for elucidating the molecular mechanisms at their basis, has resulted, over time, in the development of a huge number of liver-derived models and systems, that has not been equalled in the case of any other human organ/tissue (see Table 2).

Models	Advantages	Drawbacks	References
Human liver-derived single enzymes, supersomes, sub-cellular and organelles' fractions (cytosol, microsomes, mitochondria, S-9 fractions)	- Useful for identifying mechanisms/enzymes/ metabolism of drug- and chemical-induced hepatotoxicity - Contain a rich variety of metabolic enzymes for studying the *in vitro* metabolism of drugs - High availability - Easy to prepare, use and store - Mitochondrial dysfunctions and energy metabolism studies are allowed - Molecular/sub-cellular investigations	- Only sub-acute/acute toxicity studies - Extremely simplified models, lacking whole gene regulation systems, cell-cell interactions, bile canaliculi, transporters, cell structures and functions - For extrapolation to whole cell, all sub-cellular fractions should be tested - Low level of enzyme activity may be faced - Difficult extrapolation to whole *in vivo* organism - Lack of concordance with the *in vivo* situation (microsomes lack some phase II enzymes)	Boelsterli & Lim, 2007 Clarke & Jeffrey, 2001 Guengerich, 1996 Mae *et al.*, 2000 Rawden *et al.*, 2005
Reporter gene-based systems (mainly P450 enzymes-expressing models): recombinant hepatoma cells, liver supersomes, microsomes	- Supply drug-metabolizing or functional capacity to cellular systems lacking metabolic enzymes/ transporters - Provide information about single CYP enzymes - Readily available - All known human cytochrome P450 (CYPs) have been successfully over-expressed in genetically modified organisms	- Only sub-acute/acute toxicology studies - Lack of other phase I and phase II biotransformation enzymes - Extremely simplified model - The transduced isoform is in excess as compared to physiological concentration *in vivo*	Huang *et al.*, 2000
Single liver cells analysis	- Single cell approach of biological process - High availability of cells - Possibility to test high broad number of drugs in various culture conditions	- Very short-term studies - Sub-acute/acute toxicity studies - Need optimisation of investigation tools	O'Brien *et al.*, 2006 Xu *et al.*, 2004
Isolated hepatocytes in suspension	- Highly available - Easy-to-handle - Poor functional activity - Applicability to High-throughput screening (HTS): limited - Could support kinetic, and drug-drug interactions studies	- Short-term cell viability (2-4 hrs) - Sub-acute/acute toxicity studies - Phenotypic instability due to alteration of tissue architecture and ECM, loss of cell polarisation/organisation - Loss of cell-cell / cell-ECM interactions - High variability between batches - Absence of non-parenchymal cells	Guillouzo, 1998 Richert *et al.*, 2006
Hepatic cell lines in conventional 2D culture (examples of human-derived cell lines: HepG2, Hep3B, HepaRG, HepZ, C3A,THLE; examples of non-human hepatic cell lines: HTC, BRL3A and NRL clone 9, Fa32 and WIF-B9)	- Almost infinite capacity of proliferation - High availability - Easy-to-handle (culture, freezing, etc.) - Possibility to genetically engineer cells (Hep3B, HepaR, THLE) - Avoid repeated cell isolation - High reproducibility - Moderate cost - Applicable to HTS - Differentiated phenotype variably expressed, according to the cell line (e.g. HepG2 cells express CYP1A,	- Acute toxicity studies - Lack or limited/partial drug-metabolism capacity and other hepatic functions - Absence of non-parenchymal cells - Expression of typical phenotype, depending on culture conditions and passaging - No accurate modelling of *in vivo* hepatic phenotype (genetically instable and/or derived from malignant tissues)	Boess *et al.*, 2003 Dierickx, 2003 Guillouzo *et al.*, 2007 Jennen *et al.*, 2010 Kanebratt & Andersson, 2008 Malatesta *et al.*, 2008 Payen *et al.*, 1999

Models	Advantages	Drawbacks	References
	CYP2B, CYP3A, CYP2E, UDPGT, GST, but lack other drug metabolizing enzymes; HepRG cells express CYP1A2, CYP2B6, CYP2C9, CYP3A4, CYP2E1, GSTAs, UGT1A1, some ABC transporters, some plasma proteins, but not always in homogeneous way) - According to the cell line: metabolic profiling; kinetic studies; drug-drug interaction, mechanistic studies and short-term toxicity screening		Richert, et al., 2006 Schoonen et al., 2009 Slany et al., 2010 Werner et al., 2000 Wilkening & Bader, 2003
2D primary cultures of hepatocytes in static conditions (monotypic cultures)	- Primary human hepatocytes represent the *in vitro* model of choice for drug screening - Express most of CYP isoforms (e.g. CYP1A2, CYP2A6, CYP2B6, CYP2C9, CYP2C19, CYP2D6, CYP2E1, CYP3A4) - Express phase II biotransformation enzymes (e.g. UDPGT, SULT2A1, GST) - Easy to use and fast - Short-term preservation of cell viability, liver-specific functions and gene responsiveness - High/medium efficient cryopreservation - At high density or confluence, cell-cell contacts may be rebuilt - Reproducible method - Short-time inducibility of phase I and phase II enzymes by xenobiotics - Applicable to HTS - Could support: metabolic profiling, pharmacokinetic (ADME) and drug-drug interactions (DIDs) studies, mechanistic studies and short-term toxicity screening	- Early phenotypic alterations (about 75% of total CYP activity within the first 24 hrs)= loss of accuracy - Scarcity of human liver - Isolation is time consuming and may damage cells - Limited proliferation - Difficulty to mimic the *in vivo* microenvironment - Loss of cell polarity, tissue architecture, membrane domains - Lack of non-parenchymal cell types - Inter-donor variability (human liver) - Batch-to-batch variability of isolated hepatocytes - High influence of culture conditions on cell features - Inter-species variability	Gomez-Lechon et al., 2007 Guillouzo, 1998 Hewitt et al., 2007 Lecluyse et al., 2001
Somatic cells (trans-differentiation into hepatocytes), hepatic stem/progenitor cells	- Could express a large panel of liver-specific genes (including those involved in biotransformation processes)	- A great effort is needed to reach a fully differentiated phenotype and for use in risk assessment - Variability in the phenotype expressed by "hepatocytes"	Lee et al., 2004 Schwartz et al., 2002
2D co-cultures of liver-derived cell types (heterotypic culture, at large- or at micro-scale)	- Higher cell viability than monotypic culture (2 weeks) - Maintain some hepatic functions for longer time (plasma protein, urea secretion, lipoprotein metabolism, some CYPs) - Maintain heterotypic cell-cell interactions	- Only some liver specific functions are slightly maintained after longer time in culture (up from 7 to 15 days)	Guzzardi et al., 2009 Ijima et al., 2005 Khetani & Bhatia, 2008 Ohno et al., 2008
3D cultures of primary hepatocytes/hepatic cell lines/stem cells without (spheroids,	- Maintain more hepatic functions for longer time (up to some weeks) - A number of genes are up-regulated (albumin, transferrin, fibrinogen,	- Cell recovery is sometimes difficult - Loss of liver-specific functions (decline of some CYP activities) - In some 3D models, formation of	Chang & Hughes-Fulford, 2009 Du et al., 2008

Models	Advantages	Drawbacks	References
micromasses) or with scaffolds (micropatterned polydimethylsiloxane surfaces; nanofibrillar network; hydrogels Sandwich cultures: collagen-collagen, collagen-matrigel, alginate encapsulation, or RGD-galactose)	prothrombin, CYP1A1, CYP1A2, CYP2E1, CYP3A, etc.) - Ureagenesis varies according to the model, and may be 6-7 times as in classical 2D culture - High level of hepatic transporters - Fluidic dynamic of some bioreactor favours shear stress and support liver-specific gene expression - Improve microenvironment features - Hepatocytes are much more sensitive to some xenobiotics than in static 2D culture - After optimisation of culture and microenvironment conditions, these models could be used for chronic toxicology	necrotic cores: - According to the 3D model, specific hepatic function are maintained - Currently unsuitable for HTS (need the development of adequate methods/devices for increasing sensitivity and reliability, lowering cost and time-consuming features)	Evenou et al., 2007 Kienhuis et al., 2007 Liu Tsang et al., 2007 Maguire et al., 2007 Meng, 2010 Miranda et al., 2010 Suzuki et al., 2008 Walker & Woodrooffe, 2001
3D co-cultures of liver-derived cell types	- Longer cell viability, as compared to monotypic 3D culture (up to 57 days) - Sustain some liver-specific function from 3 days to 7 up weeks (albumin, urea secretion, expression of CYP1A1/2,CYP2B1, CYP3A) - Mimic liver cyto-organisation/cyto-orientation - Intercellular interactions and communications - Soluble factors enhance hepatocytes functions	According to culture conditions: - variable cell viability and differentiation status - need bioreactor optimisation to increase mass transfer - in situ approaches/techniques need to be developed to be applicable for HTS (see 3D monotypic cultures)	Bennett et al., 2006 Bhatia et al., 1999 Cheng et al., 2008 Leite et al., 2011 Ohno et al., 2008 Riccalton-Banks et al., 2003
Precision-cut liver slices	- Several aspects of in vivo microenvironment are preserved - Retain in vivo cyto-/histo-architecture - Acinar sub-localization of functions - Cellular heterogeneity (include non-parenchymal cells) - Expression of functional drug metabolizing enzymes (CYP1A, CYP2A, CYP2B, CYP2C and CYP 3A sub-families) and transporters - Preservation of hepatocyte polarity - Could support metabolic profiling, mechanistic studies and, less easily, toxicity screening	- Short-term viability (about 5 days) - Short-term metabolic studies (about 48 to 72 hrs) - Progressive formation of necrotic cores - Poorly amenable to HTS - Limited liver-specific functions - Scarcity of human liver donors - High intra-assay variability - Donor-to-donor variability - Hard to handle - Poorly efficient cryopreservation - Poor diffusion of drugs across the slides	Elferink et al., 2008 Krumdieck, et al., 1980 Lake et al., 1996 Schumacher et al., 2007
Isolated perfused liver (resections/whole animal liver)	- Maintenance of whole organ features and functionality (cell-cell and cell-ECM interactions, cell polarisation, cell heterogeneity, 3D organisation, zonation) - Represent the closest models mimicking in vivo situation - Allow real-time bile collection/analysis and oxygen consumption - Liver injury is reflected by LDH, AST, and ALT	- Very short-term studies are possible (2-3 hours) - Hard to handle - Expensive model - Poor reproducibility - Difficult inter-species extrapolation - Impossibility to be applied to human liver	Gores et al., 1986 şahin, 2003

Models	Advantages	Drawbacks	References
Integrated discrete multiple organ co-culture systems	- Try to re-create the organ-organ cross talks (paracrine factors) - Assessment of organ-specific toxicity - Short-term (48 hrs) assessment of the biological/toxicological effect of native drugs and their metabolites/catabolites	- Need optimisation for HTS - Biotransformation of drug need to be known earlier to optimise cell culture and spatial organisation (or determined by random positioning) - Some limitations related to the 2D configuration	Li, 2008 and 2009
Whole organism	- Maintenance of systemic interrelations, tissue integrity and normal hepatic functions (for the considered specie) - Maintenance of liver physiology - Well known and often standardized methods - Whole system inter-relation is preserved - Allow to take into account the biokinetic features of drugs/molecules, (ADME/toxicology processes are maintained)	- Ethically discussable - Need to be revised for applying the 3R's concept - Need of GPL practice - Inter-species variability and difficulty to reflect human context (human-specific metabolites, inherent sensitivity of peculiar population) = difficulty and risk of unreliability, extrapolation of results from animal to human for xenobiotic metabolism as well as target organ sensibility - In clinical trials: inter-individual variability, limitations of trial endpoint and population sampling - Expensive and time consuming - Uncontrolled sources of variability, such as housing conditions of animals, subjectivity in scoring, etc.	Li, 2004

New computational *(in silico)* models, toxicogenomics-, transcriptomics-, proteomics- and metabolomics-based models present important advantages for risk assessment, but they need adequate *in vivo* or *in vitro* models to be reliable (Cheng & Dixon, 2003; Khor *et al.*, 2006; Hunt *et al.*, 2007; Valerio, 2009; Amacher, 2010; Gómez-Lechón, *et al.*, 2010).

Table 2. Experimental approaches used for hepatic risk assessment.

The first and simplest *in vitro* liver models were optimised for studying single metabolic functions, and are based on the use of hepatic sub-cellular fractions (single enzymes, microsomes, supersomes, cytosolic fractions and mixed fractions). Although such models are easy to use, they fail in mimicking the complete and complex metabolic potential of hepatocytes, as well as intra-lobular zonal specialisation and inter-individual heterogeneity of the liver-specific cell phenotype. Not even the models based on the use of liver-derived cell lines are considered to be fully reliable, even though, for their metabolic characteristics, they are more complete than the sub-cellular fractions, and present the advantage of limitless culture time. These cell lines, generated from malignant tumours or obtained from transformed cells, present, in effect, the disadvantage of having lost the majority of their original phenotypic features.

In the same way, also engineered cells or systems (e.g. microsomes) based on reporter gene transfer have been shown to be not sufficiently reliable and informative (for more exhaustive information on the principal *in vitro* hepatic models traditionally in use, see also Brandon *et al.*, 2003, Zucco *et al.*, 2004, Gómez-Lechón *et al.*, 2007, Guillouzo & Guguen-Guillouzo, 2008).

It is now well recognised that any experimental model that has to be used for reproducing *in vitro* the function of human liver, must be developed from human hepatocytes in primary culture (Gómez-Lechón *et al.*, 2007). The scarce availability of tissue, its variable quality, and the difficulty to succeed, with the traditional techniques, in maintaining isolated hepatocytes *in vitro*, preserving their viability and functions for long-term studies, have strongly hindered the refinement of these models, limiting, in such a way, the significance of their use (Gómez-Lechón *et al.*, 2007; Guillouzo & Guguen-Guillouzo, 2008). No result worthy of further consideration has been derived from the very large number of attempts performed to get well-differentiated hepatocytes from stem precursors, either originating from the liver itself (resident hepatic progenitors), or from extra-hepatic sites (e.g. bone marrow and adipose tissue), or from mesenchymal cells, obtained in precocious phases of the development (cells from umbilical cord blood or embryonic stem cells) (Cantz *et al.*, 2008). Advantages and limits of these cells as "hepatocyte donors" are summarized in Table 3.

Cell type	Origin	Characteristics	Reference
Embryonic stem cells (ESCs)	Derived from the inner cell mass of pre-implantation-stage blastocysts	⊕ Totipotent stem cells ⊕ Self-renewal ⊕ Huge proliferative potential ⊕ High differentiation potential and plasticity ⊕ Expression of early markers of hepatic differentiation ⊕ Some mature hepatic functions are maintained ⊖ Difficulty to be regulated and maintained under controlled conditions ⊖ Risk of oncogenicity ⊖ Ethical issues ⊖ Limited availability	Agarwal *et al.*, 2008 Baharvand *et al.*, 2006 & 2008 Ishii, *et al.* 2010 Jozefczuk *et al.*, 2011 Liu T *et al.*, 2010 Rambhatla , *et al.*, 2003 Soto-Gutierrez *et al.*, 2007
Extra-hepatic adult stem cells	Bone marrow	⊕ Pluripotent stem cells ⊕ Inducible to express a number of liver-specific functions ⊖ Difficulty to reach full adult hepatocyte phenotype ⊖ Less differentiated than primary hepatocytes	Avital *et al.*, 2001 Chen *et al.*, 2006 Chivu *et al.*, 2009 Petersen *et al.*, 1999
	Adipose tissue	⊕ Pluripotent stem cells ⊕ Express to some extent specific hepatic functions ⊖ Quantitatively less differentiated than HEPG$_2$ cell line ⊖ Less differentiated than primary hepatocytes	Okura *et al.*, 2010
	Umbilical cord blood	⊕ Pluripotent stem cells ⊕ Express some hepatic markers ⊖ Further investigations are necessary to better characterize their differentiation status ⊖ Less differentiated than primary hepatocytes	Campard *et al.*, 2008 Hong *et al.*, 2005 Lee *et al.*, 2004
	Peripheral blood	⊕ CD14+ peripheral blood monocytes ⊕ Well differentiated hepatocyte-like cells (expression of a number of liver-specific functions) ⊕ Easy to obtain ⊖ Multi-laboratory investigations should be done to validate the method	Ruhnke *et al.*, 2005 Ehnert , 2008 and 2011

Cell type	Origin	Characteristics	Reference
Adult/foetal stem cells and hepatic progenitors	Liver	⊕ Multi-potent stem cells ⊕ Different adult stem cells typologies ⊖ Still difficult to use for therapeutic applications ⊖ Hardly obtainable	Dan & Yeoh, 2008 Turner, 2011
	Hepatic progenitors (usually localised in small biliary canals)	⊕ Bi-potential cells ⊕ Differentiate in both hepatocytic and biliary lineages ⊖ Low cell number (in adult liver) ⊖ Difficult proposal for human derived cells	Dan & Yeoh, 2008 Zhang *et al.*, 2008
	Foetal hepatocytes, hepatoblast precursors	⊕ Multi-potent stem cells ⊕ High proliferation rate ⊕ Exhibit some biotransformation pathways ⊕ Bi-potential plasticity ⊖ Ethical problems for human donors	Dan *et al.*, 2006, Ring *et al.*, 2010
	Somatic adult cells: hepatocytes	⊕ Temporary high differentiated phenotype ⊖ Unipotent cells ⊖ Low replication rate ⊖ Rapid cell function decrease ⊖ Low cell availability for human cells	Gomez-Lechon *et al.*, 2007
Induced pluripotent stem cells (iPS)	From connective tissues (fibroblasts or other somatic cells)	⊕ Pluripotent cells ⊕ Highly proliferative cells ⊕ Capability to differentiate into liver-specific parenchymal cells ⊕ Quite similar to hESCs ⊕ Very promising technology ⊖ Lowest replication and differentiation capability than ESCs ⊖ Immature and incomplete hepatic phenotype ⊖ Still need the optimisation of differentiating protocols ⊖ Development of iPS without virus could represent a great challenge also for therapeutic applications ⊖ Need further development of differentiating strategy (type of differentiating factor to be used, spatio-temporal release of factors), optimisation and standardisation of induction protocols and culture conditions, as well as an increase of the quality control of the final cell preparation	Takahashi *et al.*, 2007 Espejel *et al.*, 2010 Hu *et al.*, 2010 Q. Feng *et al.*, 2010 Sullivan *et al.*, 2010 H. Liu *et al.*, 2010 & 2011 Greenbaum, 2010 Si-Tayeb *et al.*, 2010
Trans-differentiated cells	Epithelial cells	⊕ Bi-potent cells ⊖ Immature cell functions are expressed	Snykers, 2007
	Pancreatic cells (healthy or tumour-derived)	⊕ Some differentiated hepatic enzymes are expressed ⊖ Difficult to propose for human-derived cells	Tosh , 2002 Burke *et al.*, 2006 and 2007

Table 3. Cell types commonly used for the design of *in vitro* hepatic models and liver tissue engineering.

The hepatocyte is a structurally complex epithelial cell and represents the major hepatic parenchymal cell type, either in terms of mass (60% of the total number of liver cells and 80% of the total volume of the organ), or for the number of functions carried out. Cholangiocytes and non-parenchymal cells [sinusoidal endothelial cells, stellate cells (fat-storing Ito cells), pit cells (intrahepatic lymphocytes), Kupffer cells, and hepatocyte precursors] influence, by their presence and activity, hepatocyte survival and function (Selden et al., 1999; Riccalton-Banks et al., 2003; Nahmias et al., 2006; Catapano & Gerlach, 2007). The extracellular matrix (ECM) represents another key component of this organ: it is peculiar by composition and structure, and it plays a determinant role in regulating hepatocyte viability, as well as other biological processes, such as development, proliferation, migration and functional activity (Selden et al., 1999; Van de Bovenkamp et al., 2007). Being functionally and structurally polarised, the hepatocyte requires, in effect, precise and specific cell-cell and cell-matrix interactions. The characteristic cyto-architecture of liver, organised as "lobular" units, entails, furthermore, a particular morphological and functional specialisation of hepatocytes, that varies with position along the liver sinusoid, from the portal triad to the central vein ("zonation") (see Fig. 1 and Fig. 3). It is now well accepted that this regional compartmentalisation of metabolic (and detoxification) functions of hepatocytes within the "acinus" is responsible for the "zone-specific" liver susceptibility to many hepatotoxic agents (Lindros et al., 1997). The hepatocellular "zonation", sustained by portocentral patterns of gene expression ("gradient" versus "compartmental" and "dynamic" versus "stable" types of zonation), is modulated by chemical gradients of oxygen, hormones, growth factors and metabolites, which are generated and maintained as a result of the specific characteristics of the ECM and of the distribution of non-parenchymal cells (Gebhardt, 1992; Christoffels et al., 1999). This specific microenvironment, dynamic, highly organised and rigidly structured, is thus fundamental for maintaining hepatic functions. It is, actually, well known, how the subversion of liver architecture produced by the alteration/destruction of the strict relationship hepatocyte-matrix and hepatocyte-non parenchymal cells, that occurs as a consequence of trauma or pathological states (e.g. fibrosis), is responsible for important negative effects on liver homeostasis and loss of functions (Selden et al., 1999; Van de Bovenkamp et al., 2007). Experimental models of liver should, therefore, take into account the strict inter-dependence between the complex histo-morphology of this organ and its functions/responses (Allen et al., 2005).

The need to preserve the original cytological and histo-architectural features of the hepatic tissue has provided the basis for attempting to develop various ex vivo hepatic models (Table 2). Among these models, the best known is the isolated and perfused organ model (Gores et al., 1986, Bessems et al., 2006). Although this model is considered to be the closest representation of the in vivo situation, its use is limited to a few hours; moreover, the necessity to employ a whole organ for each single experimental point, leads to a very broad range of variability in the results (Gores et al., 1986), and makes impossible the use of human-derived tissue. As an alternative, the model based on the culture of organ slices, obtained by particular section methods (precision-cut liver slices) has been developed. Notwithstanding this model may solve, at least partially, the problem of results' variability, it still presents, employed with the conventional culture techniques, the disadvantage of limited cells' survival (only a few days), even if slice thickness is maintained under the physical limit of diffusion of gas and nutrients (200 µm) (Fisher et al., 2001, Vickers et al., 2011). Despite the development of new dynamic culture methods (see later) renders the

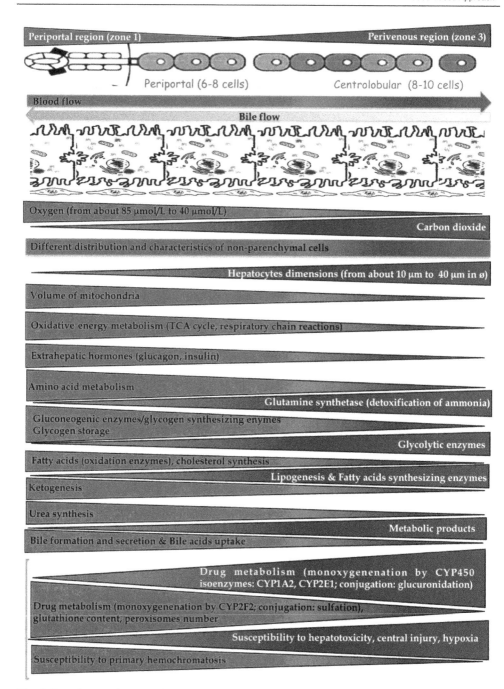

Fig. 3. Zonal specialisation of liver acinus, from periportal to centrolobular region, and different susceptibility to toxic agents.

future of this model very promising, due to the fact that, by preserving intact the original tissue microenvironment (ECM, multi-cellularity and histo-architecture), it could be very close to the liver *in vivo* (Van de Bovenkamp *et al.*, 2007), liver slices do not possess, at present, such characteristics. The more ordinary models used in the study of hepatic function, with their relative advantages/disadvantages, are illustrated in Table 2.

3. Three-dimensional liver-derived *in vitro* systems: Tissue engineering and the contribute of the new technologies

As in the case of other tissue models, it is now generally accepted that any attempt aimed at the generation of reliable and physiologically relevant *in vitro* liver analogues, should take into account the need of reproducing (or conserving) the specific characteristics of the original microenvironment typical of that organ (see above). The main features of the environmental context within which cells physiologically grow, proliferate and express their own functions, include, in addition to multiple cellularity, biochemical and mechanical properties (that are specific of each organ/tissue), also the three-dimensionality (Mazzoleni *et al.*, 2009).

Over the last few decades, it has already been widely demonstrated that, compared to the use of traditional culture techniques in monolayer (2D), three-dimensional (3D) culture methods allow researchers to generate *in vitro* tissue-derived model systems that better mimic the *in vivo* situation (Pampaloni *et al.*, 2007). Significant differences have, in fact, been demonstrated between the biological behaviour of cellular elements (hepatocytes included) maintained in culture with traditional (2D) culture methods, and that of cells kept in 3D culture (Mazzoleni *et al.*, 2009). Figure 4 presents a qualitative comparison between the most important characteristics of the different currently used liver model systems.

The importance of being able to reproduce *in vitro* the 3D specific microenvironment typical of the tissue of origin, has led to the design and development of increasingly complex and sophisticated 3D culture methods. These methods, benefiting also from the rapid development of tissue engineering techniques, have produced, especially in the case of the liver, an extremely wide variety of models (Nahmias *et al.*, 2006). In the case of the liver, due to the high structural complexity of its tissue microenvironment (see above), any attempt to apply the principles of tissue engineering aimed to generate constructs capable of reproducing, *in vitro*, the specific characteristics of the organ *in vivo*, implies to face extremely difficult technical problems, which also result from having to consider issues that must be performed on spatial and temporal scales that are "gigantic". For example: the hepatocyte can recognize the structural characteristics of the surface on which it must adhere with a threshold of nanometers in size, but it should organise itself in hierarchical structures of centimetres in size; similarly, the presence of particular molecules may alter the structural characteristics of the hepatocyte's microenvironment within a few milliseconds, while the time required for the cell to functionally adapt to these changes can take several weeks (Mitzner *et al.*, 2001).

Over the years, the research in this direction has been mainly devoted to the generation of new materials (micro- and nano-structured), which possess physical and biochemical characteristics suitable to fulfil mechanical and biological support to the physiological hepatocyte activities. In particular, also due to the contribution of the new emerging technologies, the number of liver models that have been generated within the last ten years, by using the principles of tissue engineering, has been enormous.

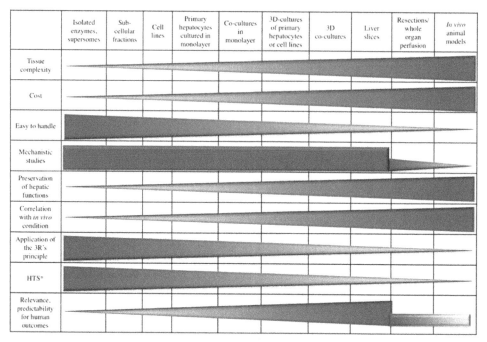

	Isolated enzymes, supersomes	Sub-cellular fractions	Cell lines	Primary hepatocytes cultured in monolayer	Co-cultures in monolayer	3D-cultures of primary hepatocytes or cell lines	3D co-cultures	Liver slices	Resections/ whole organ perfusion	*In vivo* animal models
Tissue complexity										
Cost										
Easy to handle										
Mechanistic studies										
Preservation of hepatic functions										
Correlation with *in vivo* condition										
Application of the 3R's principle										
HTS*										
Relevance, predictability for human outcomes										

Fig. 4. Comparison of the most diffused hepatic model systems. Primary hepatocytes cultured in monolayer represent the most diffused model. * HTS: suitable for high-throughput screening.

Since differentiated hepatocytes are anchorage-dependent, immotile and non-proliferating cells, the first "liver-like engineered microenvironments" had, as primary objective, to ensure well-defined characteristics of the substrates (bio/artificial matrices), in terms of architecture (nano-fibrillar), porosity (micro- and macro- scale), and biochemical composition. The products that are now available (even commercially), are hydro-gels and 3D surfaces, composed of specific constituents of original extra-cellular matrices (extractive or synthetic origin), and solid supports (micro-carriers or scaffolds, also pre-shaped), made up of porous, bio-compatible, organic or synthetic components. Examples of the sophisticated models that, for various purposes, have been obtained from primary hepatocytes, are those generated by using bio-degradable nano-structured substrates (Kim *et al.*, 1998), heat-sensitive polymers (Ohashi *et al.*, 2007), various 3D matrices (Fiegel *et al.*, 2008; ZQ. Feng *et al.*, 2010; Ghaedi *et al.*, 2012), or synthetic self-assembling hydrogels (Wang *et al.*, 2008).

The development of the micro- and nano-technologies (i.e. micro-/nano-fabrication techniques, micro-electronics and micro-fluidics), has allowed the creation of models where the cellular elements are integrated into controlled microenvironments, within which, in addition to the precise definition of the spatio-temporal signals individual cells are exposed to, it is also possible to perform the continuous multi-parameter monitoring of their biological responses ("lab-on-a-chip" devices). Representative examples of this approach, applied to cultured hepatocytes, and aimed at generating functional models of liver lobules, bile canaliculi and sinusoids, have been given, respectively, by Ho *et al.* (2006), Lee *et al.*

(2007), and, more recently, by Nakao *et al.*, 2011. Although structurally very complex and interesting, these models of "micro-structured tissue-like environments" have major drawbacks, that limit significantly their application: they lack, in effect, the complexity of original tissue-specific microenvironments, which are typical of the situation *in vivo*; moreover, they do not allow cell survival for time periods higher than several hours or days.

4. Bioreactors and relative microgravity condition

It is well known that the metabolic requirements of complex 3D cell constructs are substantially higher than those needed for the maintenance of traditional cell monolayers (2D culture) kept in liquid media under static conditions.

The first "dynamic" bioreactors were, in effect, designed in order to meet the necessity of increasing the "mass transfer" rate, for facilitating an adequate long-term supply of gases and nutrients (and the removal of metabolic waste) up to the cellular elements placed in the inner parts of complex 3D tissue explants or tissue-like constructs. Taking advantage of the great progress in the development of new technologies, and of the contribution of computational fluid dynamics, a wide array of dynamic bioreactors have been devised (from the simplest stirred- or suspension-based culture systems, to the more complex membrane-based reactors, and their more sophisticated versions, that include load-, continuously perfused-/pulsed-systems, and multi-compartmentalised bioreactors, able to generate highly controlled microenvironments) (Török *et al.*, 2001, Martin & Vermette, 2005; Catapano & Gerlach, 2007; Meuwly *et al.*, 2007, Guzzardi *et al.* 2011). However, despite all of these technological efforts, none of these bioreactors are, at present, able to provide optimal conditions for the long-term maintenance of large tissue-like masses in culture. The current generation of bioreactors was, in reality, developed for yielding large masses of cells (or cell products) for industrial or clinical applications, and not for supporting the survival or the self-assembly of multiple cell types into complex 3D tissue-like structures (Hutmacher & Singh, 2008). This applies, in particular, to the liver, a highly specialized organ, whose cellular components are extremely sensitive to even minimal environmental changes, already under physiological conditions (Nahmias *et al.*, 2006; Catapano & Gerlach, 2007).

An important aspect, essential for the appropriate choice of the specific device to use for cell/tissue culture methods, is the consideration that, even if hydrodynamic forces effectively increase mass transfer, in dynamic bioreactors for 3D culturing this effect should be achieved by considering (and balancing) the detrimental effect of turbulence and shear stress on cell survival and function. Low-shear environment and optimal mass transfer have been attained only with the introduction of the Rotary Cell Culture System (RCCS™, Synthecon, Inc.) bioreactors. This technology, fruit of N.A.S.A.'s Johnson Space Center technological research and optimised over the last ten years, has been successfully used in ground- as well as in space-based studies on a wide variety of cell types and tissues (a vast literature is available at http://www.synthecon.com). RCCS™ bioreactors provide several advantages, when compared to other available 3D culture systems (Mazzoleni & Steimberg, 2010). A comparison of the main features of various bioreactors (static or dynamic flow condition) commonly used in the foremost culture techniques is presented in Table 4.

Horizontally rotating, transparent clinostats, RCCS™ devices efficiently create a unique, highly controlled microenvironment that, by reproducing some aspects of microgravity (simulated microgravity) (Klaus, 2001; Ayyaswamy & Mukundakrishnan, 2007), guarantee the most favourable conditions for cell and tissue culturing (Schwarz *et al.*, 1992), and provide potentially powerful tools to reproduce specific 3D tissue morphogenesis (Mazzoleni *et al.*, 2009). Complex tissue-like 3D constructs, different cell types from various origins and various intact tissue explants have been demonstrated, by our group and others, to be kept efficiently in culture by these bioreactors, even for long periods of time (Unsworth & Lelkes, 1998; Hammond & Hammond, 2001; Vunjak-Novakovic *et al.*, 2002; Nickerson *et al.*, 2007; Cosmi *et al.*, 2009; Steimberg *et al.*, 2009, Steimberg *et al.*, 2010; Mazzoleni *et al.*, 2011).

Figure 5 shows selected examples of RCCS™-based tissue culture methods, developed and optimised by our group, and their advantages.

	Shear stress	Mass transfer (gas/nutrient supply; waste removal)	Dimensionality	Adequate for co-culture	Maintenance of liver- specific phenotype
Static 2D culture (monolayer)	No	Adequate	2D	Moderately	Few hours/ days
Static 2D culture (on biosynthetic matrices)	No	Limited	3D (limited)	Moderately	Few days/weeks
Roller bottles	Moderate	Moderate	2D	Poorly	Few days
Spinner flasks	High	High	3D (very limited)	Poorly	Few days/weeks
Microfluidic bioreactors	Moderate/ High	High	2D/ 3D	Moderately	Few days/weeks
Perfused bioreactors	High	High	3D (very limited)	No	Few weeks
Zonation-based devices	High	Optimal	3D	To some extent	Several days
Hollow fiber bioreactors	Low	High	3D (very limited)	To some extent	Some days/ few weeks
RCCS™ bioreactors	Low	Optimal	3D	Yes	Some weeks

Table 4. Static and dynamic bioreactor platforms used in 2D and 3D culture methods.

Even in the case of liver models, it has been demonstrated how these bioreactors allow for the maintenance of isolated human primary liver cells and tissue explants *in vitro*, under conditions that preserve their viability and differentiated functional characteristics, even for long periods (several weeks). Khaoustov *et al.* (1999) have, for example, showed that human hepatocytes, adherent on small biodegradable substrates, were able to survive for 60 days, form specific junctional complexes and structures similar to bile canaliculi, and retain the ability to biosynthesize proteins. The microgravity-based culture conditions generated by the RCCS™ bioreactor have also proved to ensure the long-term survival and preservation of the differentiated metabolic functions in the case of isolated hepatocytes in monotypic 3D culture (cellular spheroids) (Dabos, 2001), in co-culture with endothelial cells (heterotypic cultures), and in the more complex case of liver tissue homogenates, as well (Yoffe, 1999). Similar observations have also been reported by our group, proving that, under microgravity conditions, primary isolated hepatocytes organize themselves autonomously into multicellular spheroids, with properties similar, for many aspects, to normal liver cells *in vivo* (Mazzoleni *et al.*, 2008). Finally, Wurm *et al.* (2009) have also described an interesting application of the RCCS™ technology for its possible use in the clinical field, as an alternative to conventional models of bioartificial liver (BAL).

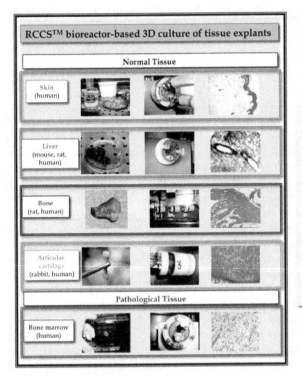

Fig. 5. Examples of RCCS™-based tissue culture methods, developed and optimised by our group, and their advantages.

5. Conclusions

The 3D culture methods based on the use of the dynamic RCCS™ bioreactor demonstrates that they can guarantee the best conditions for generating *in vitro* microenvironments suitable for the long-term maintenance of viable liver-derived parenchymal cells and tissue explants. These techniques enable, moreover, to preserve some of the native and typical morpho-functional characteristics of the organ *in vivo*. For these reasons, the RCCS™-based 3D culture methods illustrated in this chapter present, in the current scientific context, the most promising prospect for the development of physiologically significant liver models, which may, in the future, be usefully employed in basic and applied research, in pharmaco-toxicology, risk assessment, and in clinical fields. Remarkably, the rapid progress in the development of new experimental protocols and analytical methods, together with the possibility of using this innovative microgravity-based culture technology for the development of liver-derived complementary *in vitro* models, based on the use of human isolated cells or intact tissue explants (healthy or pathological), could, indeed, open new perspectives for the study of important (and still unknown) aspects of the patho-physiology (functions and responses) of this complex organ. Once optimised (and validated), these *in vitro* (cell-based) and *ex-vivo* (tissue-based) human liver models should also allow new applications in the field of pharmaco-toxicology and risk assessment, and, in addition, could permit to reduce the need of experimental animals. By mimicking human liver functions and responses, these models could, in effect, be used either for studying mechanisms of toxicity (identification of critical toxicological pathways/targets), or, if adequately optimised, for screening purposes (Blaauboer, 2008).

This is in line with the declared policies of the European Union (EU) and of the United States (US), which solicit more innovative approaches to toxicity testing and the reduction of animal-based studies, as it is well expressed, for example, by EU legislation (7th Amending Directive 2003/15/EC to Council Directive 76/768/EEC on Cosmetics; REACH Regulation on Chemicals and their safe use - EC 1907/2006, Council Regulation n.440/2008 on dangerous substances, and Directive 2010/63/EU on the protection of animals used for scientific purposes) (Lilienblum *et al.*, 2008; Hartung, 2010), and by the 2007 landmark report of the US National Academy of Sciences "Toxicity Testing in the 21st century. A vision and a strategy" (NRC, 2007). The NCR 2007 report emphasizes the need of replacing traditional animal-based studies with innovative testing strategies (physiologically relevant *in vitro* assays and specific *in silico* models), which, taking advantage of new advances in scientific knowledge and new technologies, could improve real exposure measurement and human health risk assessment. The report envisions a shift of the traditional paradigm of toxicology from the measurement of apical endpoints in animal models, to the proper understanding of primary toxic mechanisms ("toxicity pathways") in humans and use of computational modelling techniques (*"in silico* methods"). This vision has generated various research initiatives and several on-going projects, such as the HESI "Risk Assessment in the 21st Century" Project (RISK21) and the US Environmental Protection Agency (EPA)'s ToxCast™ program (Dix *et al.*, 2007; US EPA, 2009), aimed at advancing toxicology strategies in EU and US (Vanhaeke *et al.*, 2009; Stephens *et al.*, 2012). According to NRC 2007 vision, predictive models that need to be developed, should be based on the identification, analysis and modelling of pathways involved in human cellular responses during the transition from physiological to pathological status in response to toxicants (US EPA, 2009). Innovative tissue-specific *in vitro* models (such as the 3D RCSS™-based liver models described in this chapter can be considered), are intended to identify and evaluate key toxicity pathways perturbations (NCR, 2007), in order to create the knowledge base required to develop *in vitro* and *in silico* pathway assay test systems relevant to human risk assessment (Stephens *et al.*, 2012). The specific interest that these 3D liver models present within this new vision in toxicological risk assessment is clearly highlighted by the US EPA Strategic Plan for the Evaluation of the Toxicity of Chemicals (US EPA, 2009), in several parts of the document and, namely, when it refers to the importance of preserving the original 3D tissue-specific heterogeneous microenvironment for improving the predictive potential of *in vitro* systems (*"Some toxicities are manifest only when multiple cell types and specific cell-cell interactions are present. Other toxicities may be dependent upon tissue geometry and 3D architecture. Examples include signalling between hepatocytes and Kupffer cells, or the many forms of signalling between epithelial and mesenchymal cells.")* (US EPA, 2009).

Ultimately, microgravity-based 3D culture methods could lead to the development of new devices, suitable to support, from the clinical point of view, the liver's essential functions (e.g. new-concept "bio-artificial" livers), or lead to the design of innovative protocols for the autologous transplantation of normal or engineered hepatocytes, in order to counteract liver disorders (e.g. those caused by specific enzymatic defects).

6. Acknowledgments

The authors are grateful to Dr. Nathalie Rochet (University of Nice "Sophia-Antipolis", CNRS, UFR of Medicine, France) for the fruitful scientific discussion and the critical reading of the manuscript, and to Dr. Richard Fry (Cellon S.A., Luxembourg), for his interest in our work, and for his kind and constant help in exploring the possibilities of the 3D culture in microgravity.

This work has been partly supported by European Union grants EC Biotechnology BIO4-CT-97-2148 ("Development of 3D *in vitro* models of human tissues for pharmaco-toxicological applications") and LSHB-CT-2006-037168 ["Development of 3D *in vitro* models of estrogen-reporter mouse tissues for the pharmaco-toxicological analysis of estrogen receptors-interacting compounds – (ER-ICs)", EXERA project], and by funds of the University of Brescia.

7. References

Agarwal, S., Holton, KL. & Lanza, R. (2008). Efficient differentiation of functional hepatocytes from human embryonic stem cells. *Stem Cells,* Vol. 26, No. 5, (May 2008), pp. 1117–1127, ISSN 1549-4918

Allen, JW., Khetani, SR. & Bhatia, SN. (2005). *In vitro* zonation and toxicity in hepatocyte bioreactor. *Toxicological Sciences,* Vol. 84, No. 1, (March 2005), pp. 110-119, ISSN 1096-0929

Amacher, DE. (2010). The discovery and development of proteomic safety biomarkers for the detection of drug-induced liver toxicity. *Toxicology and Applied Pharmacology,* Vol. 245, No. 1, (May 2010), pp. 134-142, ISSN 1096-0333

Arias, I., Wolkoff, A., Boyer, J., Shafritz, D., Fausto, N., Alter, H. & Cohen, D. (2009). *The Liver: Biology and Pathobiology,* 5th Edition. John Wiley & Sons, Inc.; ISBN: 978-0-470-72313-5, Hoboken , U.S.A.

Avital, I., Inderbitzin, D., Aoki, T., Tyan, DB., Cohen, AH., Ferraresso, C., Rozga, J., Arnaout, WS. & Demetriou, AA. (2001). Isolation, Characterization, and Transplantation of Bone Marrow-Derived Hepatocyte Stem Cells. *Biochemical and Biophysical Research Communications,* (October 2001), Vol. 288, No. 1, pp. 156–164, ISSN 1090-2104

Ayyaswamy, PS. & Mukundakrishnan, K. (2007). Optimal conditions for simulating microgravity employing NASA designed rotating wall vessels. *Acta Astronautica,* Vol. 60, No. 4-7, (February-April 2007), pp. 397-405, ISSN 0094-5765

Baharvand, H., Hashemi, SM., Kazemi Ashtiani, S. & Farrokhi, A. (2006). Differentiation of human embryonic stem cells into hepatocytes in 2D and 3D culture systems *in vitro*.

The International Journal of Developmental Biology, Vol. 50, No. 7, pp. 645-652, ISSN 1696-3547

Baharvand, H., Hashemi, SM. & Shahsavani, M. (2008). Differentiation of human embryonic stem cells into functional hepatocyte-like cells in a serum-free adherent culture condition. *Differentiation,* Vol. 76, No. 5, (May 2008), pp. 465–477, ISSN 1432-0436

Bennett, TRJ., Thomson, B. & Shakesheff, KM. (2006). Hepatic stellate cells on poly (DL-lactic acid) surfaces control the formation of 3D hepatocyte co-culture aggregates *in vitro.* *European Cells & Materials,* Vol. 11, (January 2006), pp. 16-26, ISSN 1473-2262

Bessems, M., 't Hart, NA., Tolba, R., Doorschodt, BM., Leuvenink, HG., Ploeg, RJ., Minor, T. & van Gulik, TM. (2006). The isolated perfused rat liver: standardization of a time-honoured model. *Laboratory Animals,* Vol. 40, No. 3, (July 2006), pp. 236-246, ISSN 1758-1117

Bhatia, SN., Balis, UJ., Yarmush, ML. & Toner, M. (1999). Effect of cell–cell interactions in preservation of cellular phenotype: cocultivation of hepatocytes and nonparenchymal cells. *FASEB Journal,* Vol. 13, No. 14, (November 1999), pp. 1883–1900, ISSN 1530-6860

Blaauboer, BJ. (2008). The contribution of *in vitro* toxicity data in hazard and risk assessment: current limitations and future perspectives. *Toxicology Letters,* Vol. 180, No. 2, (August 2008), pp. 81-84, ISSN 1879-3169

Boelsterli, UA. & Lim, PL. (2007). Mitochondrial abnormalities-a link to idiosyncratic drug hepatotoxicity? *Toxicology and Applied Pharmacology,* Vol. 220, No. 1., (April 2007), pp. 92-107, ISSN 1096-0333.

Boess, F., Kamber, M., Romer, S., Gasser, R., Muller, D., Albertini S. & Suter L. (2003). Gene expression in two hepatic cell lines, cultured primary hepatocytes, and liver slices compared to the *in vivo* liver gene expression in rats: possible implications for toxicogenomics use of in vitro systems. *Toxicological Sciences,* Vol. 73, No. 2, (June 2003), pp. 386–402, ISSN 1096-0929

Brandon, EFA., Raap, CD., Meijerman, I., Beijnen, JH. & Shellens, JHM. (2003). An update on *in vitro* test methods in human hepatic drug biotransformation research: pros and cons. *Toxicology and Applied Pharmacology,* Vol. 189, No. 3, (June 2003), pp. 233-246, ISSN 1096-0333.

Burke, ZD., Shen, CN., Ralphs, KL. & Tosh, D. (2006). Characterization of liver function in transdifferentiated hepatocytes. *Journal of Cellular Physiology,* Vol. 206, No. 1, (January 2006), pp.147–159, ISSN 1097-4652

Burke, ZD., Thowfeequ, S., Peran, M. & Tosh, D. (2007). Stem cells in the adult pancreas and liver. *The Biochemical Journal,* Vol. 404, No. 2, (June 2007), pp.169–178, ISSN 1470-8728

Cantz, T., Manns, MP. & Ott, M. (2008). Stem cells in liver regeneration and therapy. *Cell and Tissue Research,* Vol. 331, No. 1, (January 2008), pp. 271-282, ISSN1432-0878

Campard, D., Lysy, PA., Najimi, M. & Sokal, EM. (2008). Native umbilical cord matrix stem cells express hepatic markers and differentiate into hepatocyte-like cells. *Gastroenterology* , Vol. 34, No. 3, (March 2008), pp. 833–848, ISSN 1528-0012

Catapano, G. & Gerlach, JC. (2007). Bioreactors for Liver Tissue Engineering. In: *Topics in Tissue Engineering.* Ashammakhi N., Reis R., Chiellini E. Vol. 3, pp. 1-42, retrieved from http://www.oulu.fi/spareparts/ebook_topics_in_t_e_vol3/abstracts/catapano_01.pdf

Chang, TT. & Hughes-Fulford, M. (2009). Monolayer and Spheroid Culture of Human Liver Hepatocellular Carcinoma Cell Line Cells Demonstrate Distinct Global Gene Expression Patterns and Functional Phenotypes. *Tissue Engineering: Part A*, Vol. 15, No. 3, (March 2009), pp. 559-567, ISSN 1557-8690

Chen, Y., Dong, X-J., Zhang, G-R., Shao, J-Z. & Xiang, L-X. (2006). Transdifferentiation of mouse BM cells into hepatocyte-like cells. *Cytotherapy* Vol. 8, No. 4, pp. 381–389, ISSN 1477-2566

Cheng, A. & Dixon, SL. (2003). *In silico* models for the prediction of dose-dependent human hepatotoxicity. *Journal of Computer-Aided Molecular Design*, Vol. 17, No. 12, (December 2003), pp. 811–823, ISSN 1573-4951

Cheng, N., Wauthier, E. & Reid, LM. (2008). Mature human hepatocytes from ex vivo differentiation of alginate-encapsulated hepatoblasts. *Tissue engineering: Part A*, Vol. 14, No. 1, (January 2008), pp. 1-7, ISSN 1937-335X

Chivu, M., Dima, SO., Stancu, CI., Dobrea, C., Uscatescu, V., Necula, LG., Bleotu, C., Tanase, C., Albulescu, R., Ardeleanu, C. & Popescu, I. (2009). *In vitro* hepatic differentiation of human bone marrow mesenchymal stem cells under differential exposure to liver-specific factors. *Translational Research*, Vol. 154, No. 3, (September 2009), pp. 122-132, ISSN 1931-5244

Clarke, S.E. & Jeffrey, P. (2001). Utility of metabolic stability screening: comparison of *in vitro* and *in vivo* clearance. *Xenobiotica*, Vol. 31, No. 8-9, (August-September 2001), pp. 591-598, ISSN 1366-5928

Conti, F. (2005). *Fisiologia Medica*, Edi-Ermes, ISBN 9788870513479, Milano, Italy

Cosmi, F., Steimberg, N., Dreossi, D. & Mazzoleni, G. (2009). Structural analysis of rat bone explants kept *in vitro* in simulated microgravity conditions. *Journal of the Mechanical Behavior of Biomedical Materials*, Vol. 2, No. 2, (April 2009), pp. 164-172, ISSN 1878-0180

Christoffels, VM., Sassi, H., Ruijter, JM., Moorman, AF., Grange, T. & Lamers, WH. (1999). A mechanistic model for the development and maintenance of portocentral gradients in gene expression in the liver. *Hepatology*, Vol. 29, No. 4, (April 1999), pp. 1180-1192, ISSN 1527-3350

Dabos, K., Nelson, LJ., Bradnock, TJ., Parkinson, JA., Sadler, IH., Hayes, PC. & Plevris, JN. (2001). The simulated microgravity environment maintains key metabolic functions and promotes aggregation of primary porcine hepatocytes. *Biochimica et Biophysica Acta*, Vol. 1526, No. 2, (May 2001), pp. 119-130, ISSN 0006-3002

Dan, YY., Riehle, KJ., Lazaro, C., Teoh, N., Haque, J., Campbell, JS. & Fausto, N. (2006). Isolation of multipotent progenitor cells from human fetal liver capable of differentiating into liver and mesenchymal lineages. *Proceedings of the National Academy of Sciences of the United States of America*, Vol. 103, No. 26, (June 2006), pp. 9912-9917, ISSN 1091-6490

Dan, YY. & Yeoh, GC. (2008). Liver stem cells: A scientific and clinical perspective. *Journal of Gastroenterology and Hepatology*, (May 2008), Vol. 23, No. 5, pp. 687–698, ISSN 1440-1746

Dierickx, PJ. (2003). Evidence for delayed cytotoxicity effects following exposure of rat hepatoma-derived Fa32 cells: implications for predicting human acute toxicity. *Toxicology in Vitro*, Vol. 17, No. 5-6, (October-December 2003), pp. 797–801, ISSN 1879-3177

Dix, DJ., Houck, KA., Martin, MT., Richard, AM., Setzer, RW. & Kavlock, RJ. (2007). The ToxCast program for prioritizing toxicity testing of environmental chemicals. *Toxicological Sciences*, Vol. 95, No.1, (January 2007), pp. 5-12, ISSN 1096-0929

Du, Y., Han, R., Wen, F., Ng San San, S., Xia, L., Wohland, T., Leo, HL. & Yu, H. (2008). Synthetic sandwich culture of 3D hepatocyte monolayer. *Biomaterials, Vol.* 29, No. 3, (January 2008), pp. 290-301, ISSN 1878-5905

Ehnert, S., Nussler, AK., Lehmann, A. & Dooley, S. (2008). Blood monocyte-derived neohepatocytes as in vitro test system for drug metabolism. *Drug Metabolism and Disposition : The Biological Fate of Chemicals,* Vol. 36, No. 9, (September 2008), pp. 1922-1929, ISSN 1521-009

Ehnert, S., Schyschka, L., Noss, A., Knobeloch, D., Kleeff, J., Büchler, P., Gillen, S., Stöckle, U., Burkhart, J., Fabian, E. & Nussler, AK. (2011). Further characterization of autologous NeoHepatocytes for *in vitro* toxicity testing. *Toxicology in Vitro,* (September 2011), Vol. 25, No. 6, pp. 1203-1208, ISSN 1879-3177

Elferink, MG., Olinga, P., Draaisma, AL., Merema, MT., Bauerschmidt, S., Polman, J., Schoonen, WG. & Groothuis, GM. (2008). Microarray analysis in rat liver slices correctly predicts in vivo hepatotoxicity. *Toxicology and Applied Pharmacology,* Vol. 229, No. 3, (June 2008), pp. 300-309, ISSN 1096-0333

Espejel, S., Roll, GR., McLaughlin, KJ., Lee, AY., Zhang, JY., Laird, DJ., Okita, K., Yamanaka, S. & Willenbring, H. (2010). Induced pluripotent stem cell–derived hepatocytes have the functional and proliferative capabilities needed for liver regeneration in mice. *The Journal of Clinical Investigation*, Vol. 120, No. 9, pp. 3120–3126, ISSN 1558-8238

Evenou, F., Fujii, T. & Sakai, Y. (2007). Liver cells culture on three-dimensional micropatterned polydimethylsiloxane surfaces. *Alternatives to Animal Testing and EXperimentation* (ALTEX), Vol. 14, (August 2007), pp. 21-25, ISSN 1344-0411

Feng, ZQ., Leach, MK., Chu, XH., Wang, YC., Tian, T., Shi, XL., Ding, YT. & Gu ZZ. (2010). Electrospun chitosan nanofibers for hepatocyte culture. *Journal of Biomedical Nanotechnology*, Vol. 6, No. 6, (December 2010), pp. 658-666, ISSN 1550-7041

Feng, Q., Lu, SJ., Klimanskaya, I., Gomes, I., Kim, D., Chung, Y., Honig, GR., Kim, KS. & Lanza, R. (2010). Hemangioblastic derivatives from human induced pluripotent stem cells exhibit limited expansion and early senescence. *Stem Cells*, Vol. 28, No. 4., (April 2010), pp. 704–712, ISSN 1549-4918

Fiegel, HC., Kaufmann, PM., Bruns, H., Kluth, D., Horch, RA., Vacanti, JP. & Kneser, U. (2008). Hepatic tissue engineering: from transplantation to customized cell-based liver directed therapies from the laboratory. *Journal of Cellular and Molecular Medicine,* Vol. 12, No. 1, (January-February 2008), pp. 56-66, ISSN 1582-4934

Fisher, RL., Ulreich, JB., Nakazato, PZ. & Brendel, K. (2001). Histological and biochemical evaluation of precision cut liver slices. *Toxicology Mechanisms and Methods*, Vol. 11, No. 2, (April 2001), pp. 59-71, ISSN 1537-6524

Gebhardt, R. (1992). Metabolic zonation of the liver: regulation and implications for liver function. *Pharmacology and Therapeutics*, Vol. 53, No. 3, pp. 275-354, ISSN 1879-016

Ghaedi, M., Soleimani, M., Shabani, I., Duan, Y. & Lotfi, AS. (2012). Hepatic differentiation from human mesenchymal stem cells on a novel nanofiber scaffold. *Cellular Molecular Biology Letters*, Vol. 7, No. 1, (March 2012), pp. 89-106, ISSN 1689-1392

Gómez-Lechón, MJ., Lahoz, A., Gombau, L., Castell, JV. & Donato, MT. (2010). *In Vitro* evaluation of potential hepatotoxicity induced by drugs. *Current Pharmaceutical Design*, Vol. 16, No. 17, (June 2010), pp. 1963-1977, ISSN 1873-4286

Gómez-Lechón, MJ., Castell, JV. & Donato, MT. (2007). Hepatocytes – the choice to investigate drug metabolism and toxicity in man: *In vitro* variability as a reflection of *in vivo. Chemico-Biological Interactions*, Vol. 168, No. 1, (May 2007), pp. 30-50, ISSN 1872-7786

Gores, GJ., Kost, LJ. & LaRusso, NF. (1986). The isolated perfused rat liver: conceptual and practical considerations. *Hepatology*, Vol. 6, No. 3, (May-June 1986), pp. 511-517, ISSN 1527-3350

Greenbaum, LE. (2010) From skin cells to hepatocytes: advances in application of iPS cell technology. *The Journal of Clinical Investigation*, Vol. 120, No. 9, (September 2010), pp. 3102–3105, ISSN 1558-8238

Guengerich, FP. (1996). *In vitro* techniques for studying drug metabolism. *Journal of Pharmacokinetics and Biopharmaceutics*, Vol. 24, No. 5, (October 1996), pp. 521–533, ISSN 0090-466

Guillouzo, A. (1998). Liver cell models in *in vitro* toxicology. *Environmental Health Perspectives*, Vol. 106, No. Suppl.2, (April 1998), pp. 511–532, ISSN 1552-9924

Guillouzo, A., Corlu, A., Aninat, C., Glaise, D., Morel, F. & Guguen-Guillouzo, C. (2007). The human hepatoma HepaRG cells: A highly differentiated model for studies of liver metabolism and toxicity of xenobiotics. *Chemico-Biological Interactions*, Vol. 168, No. 1, (May 2007), pp. 66–73, ISSN 1872-7786

Guillouzo, A. & Guguen-Guillouzo, C. (2008). Evolving concepts in liver tissue modelling and implications for in vitro toxicology. *Expert Opinion on Drug Metabolism and Toxicology*, Vol. 4, No. 10, (October 2008), pp. 1279-1294, ISSN 1744-7607

Guzzardi, MA., Vozzi, F. & Ahluwalia, AD. (2009). Study of the Crosstalk Between Hepatocytes and Endothelial Cells Using a Novel Multicompartmental Bioreactor: A Comparison Between Connected Cultures and Cocultures. *Tissue Engineering: Part A*, Vol. 15, No. 11, (November 2009), pp. 3635-3644, ISSN 1937-335X

Guzzardi, MA., Domenici, C. & Ahluwalia, A. (2011). Metabolic control through hepatocyte and adipose tissue cross-talk in a multicompartmental modular bioreactor. *Tissue Engineering: Part A*, Vol. 17, No. 11-12, (June 2011), pp. 1635-1642, ISSN 1937-335X

Hammond, TG. & Hammond, JM. (2001). Optimized suspension culture: the rotating-wall vessel. *American Journal of Physiology: Renal Physiology*, Vol. 281, No. 1, (July 2001), pp. 12-25, ISSN 1522-1466

Hartung, T. (2010). Comparative analysis of the revised Directive 2010/63/EU for the protection of laboratory animals with its predecessor 86/609/EEC – a t4 report. *Alternatives to Animal Experimentation*, Vol. 27, No.4, pagg. 285-303, ISSN 1868-596X

Hewitt, NJ., Lechón, MJ., Houston, JB., Hallifax, D., Brown, HS., Maurel, P., Kenna, JG., Gustavsson, L., Lohmann, C., Skonberg, C., Guillouzo, A., Tuschl, G., Li, AP., LeCluyse, E., Groothuis, GM. & Hengstler, JG. (2007). Primary hepatocytes: current understanding of the regulation of metabolic enzymes and transporter proteins, and pharmaceutical practice for the use of hepatocytes in metabolism, enzyme induction, transporter, clearance, and hepatotoxicity studies. *Drug Metabolism Reviews*, Vol. 39, No. 1, pp. 159–234, ISSN 1097-9883

Ho, CT., Lin, RZ., Chang, WY., Chang, HY. & Liu, CH. (2006). Rapid heterogeneous liver-cell on-chip patterning via the enhanced field-induced dielectrophoresis trap. *Lab on a Chip*, Vol. 6, No. 6, (June 2006), pp. 724-734, ISSN 1473-0189

Hong, SH., Gang, EJ., Jeong, JA., Ahn, C., Hwang, SH., Yang, IH., Park, HK., Han, H. & Kim, H. (2005). *In vitro* differentiation of human umbilical cord blood-derived mesenchymal stem cells into hepatocyte-like cells. *Biochemical and Biophysical Research Communications*, Vol. 330, No. 4, (May 2005), pp. 1153-1161, ISSN 1090-2104

Houck, KA. & Kavlock, RJ. (2008). Understanding mechanisms of toxicity: insights from drug discovery research. *Toxicology and Applied Pharmacology*, Vol. 227, No. 2, (March 2008), pp. 163-178, ISSN 1096-0333

Hu, BY., Weick, JP., Yu, J., Ma, LX., Zhang, XQ., Thomson, JA. & Zhang, SC. (2010). Neural differentiation of human induced pluripotent stem cells follows developmental principles but with variable potency. *Proceedings of the National Academy of Sciences of the United States of America*, Vol. 107, No. 9, (March 2010), pp. 4335–4340, ISSN 1091-6490

Huang, Z., Roy, P. & Waxman, DJ. (2000). Role of human liver microsomal CYP3A4 and CYP2B6 in catalyzing N-dechloroethylation of cyclophosphamide and ifosfamide. *Biochemical Pharmacology*, Vol. 59, No. 8, (April 2000), pp. 961-972, ISSN 1873-2968

Hunt, CA., Yan, L., Ropella, GEP., Park, S., Sheikh-Bahaei, S. & Roberts, MS. (2007). The multiscale *in silico* liver. *Journal of Critical Care*, Vol. 22, No. 4, (December 2007), pp. 348-349, ISSN 1557-8615

Hutmacher, DW. & Singh, H. (2008). Computational fluid dynamics for improved bioreactor design and 3D culture. *Trends in Biotechnology*, Vol. 26, No. 4, (April 2008), pp. 166-172, ISSN 1879-3096

Ijima, H., Murakami, S., Matsuo, T., Takei, T., Ono, T. & Kawakami, K. (2005). Enhancement of liver-specific functions of primary rat hepatocytes co-cultured with bone marrow cells on tissue culture-treated polystyrene surfaces. *Journal of Artificial Organs*, Vol. 8, No. 2, pp. 104-109, ISSN 1619-0904

Ishii, T., Yasuchika, K., Fukumitsu, K., Kawamoto, T., Kawamura-Saitoh, M., Amagai, Y., Ikai, I., Uemoto, S., Kawase, E., Suemori, H. & Nakatsuji, N. (2010). *In vitro* hepatic maturation of human embryonic stem cells by using a mesenchymal cell line derived from murine fetal livers. *Cell and Tissue Research*, Vol. 339, No. 3, (March 2010), pp. 505–512, ISSN 1432-0878

Jennen, DG., Magkoufopoulou, C., Ketelslegers, HB., van Herwijnen, MH., Kleinjans, JC., & van Delft, JH. (2010). Comparison of HepG2 and HepaRG by whole-genome gene expression analysis for the purpose of chemical hazard identification. *Toxicological Sciences*, Vol. 115, No. 1, (May 2010), pp. 66-79, ISSN 1096-0929

Jozefczuk, J., Prigione, A., Chavez, L. & Adjaye, J. (2011). Comparative analysis of human embryonic stem cell and induced pluripotent stem cell-derived hepatocyte-like cells reveals current drawbacks and possible strategies for improved differentiation. *Stem Cells and Development*, Vol. 20, No. 7, (July 2011), pp. 1259-1275, ISSN 1557-8534

Kanebratt, KP. & Andersson, TB. (2008). Evaluation of HepaRG cells as an *in vitro* model for human drug metabolism studies. *Drug Metabolism and Disposition*, Vol. 36, No. 7, (July 2008), pp. 1444-1452, ISSN 1521-009X

Khaoustov, VI., Darlington, GJ., Soriano, HE., Krishnan, B., Risen, D., Pellis, NR. & Yoffe, B. (1999). Induction of Three-Dimensional Assembly of Human Liver Cells by Simulated Microgravity. *In vitro Cellular and Developmental Biology - Animal*, Vol. 35, No. 9, (October 1999), pp. 501-509, ISSN 1543-706

Khetani, SR. & Bhatia, SN. (2008). Microscale culture of human liver cells for drug development. *Nature Biotechnology*, Vol .26, No. 1, (January 2008), pp. 120-126, ISSN 1546-1696

Khor, TO., Ibrahim, S. & Kong, AN. (2006). Toxicogenomics in drug discovery and drug development: Potential applications and future challenges. *Pharmaceutical Research*, Vol. 23, No. 8, (August 2006), pp. 1659-1664, ISSN 1573-904

Kienhuis, A.S., Wortelboer, H.M., Maas, W.J., van Herwijnen, M., Kleinjans, J.C.S., van Delft, J.H.M. & Stierum, R.H. (2007). A sandwich-cultured rat hepatocyte system with increased metabolic competence evaluated by gene expression profiling. *Toxicology in Vitro*, Vol. 21, No. 5, (August 2007), pp. 892–901, ISSN 1879-3177

Kim, SS., Utsunomiya, H., Koski, JA., Wu, BM., Cima, MJ., Sohn, J., Mukai, K., Griffith, LG. & Vacanti, JP. (1998). Survival and function of hepatocytes on a novel three-dimensional synthetic biodegradable polymer scaffold with an intrinsic network of channels. *Annals of Surgery*, Vol. 228, No. 1, (July 1998), pp. 8-13, ISSN 1528-1140

Klaus, DM. (2001). Clinostats and bioreactors. *Gravitational and Space Biology Bulletin*, Vol. 14, No. 2, (June 2001), pp. 55-64, ISSN 1089-988

Krumdieck, CL., dos Santos, JE. & Ho, KJ. (1980). A new instrument for the rapid preparation of tissue slices. *Analytical Biochemistry*, Vol. 104, No. 1, (May 1980), pp. 118–123, ISSN 1096-0309

Lake, BG., Charzat, C., Tredger, JM., Renwick, AB., Beamand, JA. & Price, R.J. (1996). Induction of cytochrome P450 isoenzymes in cultured precision-cut rat and human liver slices. *Xenobiotica*, Vol. 26, No. 3, (March 1996), pp. 297–306, ISSN 1366-5928

Lecluyse, EL. (2001). Human hepatocyte culture systems for the *in vitro* evaluation of cytochrome P450 expression and regulation. *European Journal of Pharmaceutical Sciences*, Vol. 13, No. 4, (July 2001), pp. 343-368, ISSN 1879-0720

Lee, KD., Kuo, TK., Whang-Peng, J., Chung, YF., Lin, CT., Chou, SH., Chen, JR., Chen, YP. & Lee, OK. (2004). *In vitro* hepatic differentiation of human mesenchymal stem cells. *Hepatology*, Vol. 40, No. 6, (December 2004), pp. 1275-1284, ISSN 1527-3350

Lee, PJ., Hung, PJ. & Lee, LP. (2007). An artificial liver sinusoid with a microfluidic endothelial-like barrier for primary hepatocyte culture. *Biotechnology and Bioengineering*, Vol. 97, No. 5, (August 2007), pp. 1340-1346, ISSN 1097-0290

Leite, SB., Teixeira, AP., Miranda, JP., Tostões, RM., Clemente, JJ., Sousa, MF., Carrondo, MJT. & Alves, PM. (2011). Merging bioreactor technology with 3D hepatocyte-fibroblast culturing approaches: Improved *in vitro* models for toxicological applications. *Toxicology in Vitro*, Vol. 25, No. 4, (June 2011), pp. 825–832, ISSN 1879-3177

Li, AP. (2004). Accurate prediction of human drug toxicity: a major challenge in drug development. *Chemico-Biological Interactions*, Vol. 150, No. 1, (November 2004), pp. 3–7, ISSN 1872-7786

Li, AP. (2008). *In vitro* evaluation of human xenobiotic toxicity: scientific concepts and the novel integrated discrete multiple cell coculture (IdMOC) technology. *Alternatives to Animal Experimentation*, Vol. 25, No. 1, pp. 43-49, ISSN 1868-596

Li, AP. (2009). The Use of the Integrated Discrete Multiple Organ Co- culture (IdMOC®) System for the Evaluation of Multiple Organ Toxicity. *Alternatives to Laboratory Animals*, Vol. 37, No. 4, (September 2009), pp. 377–385, ISSN 0261-1929

Lilienblum, W., Dekant, W., Foth, H., Gebel, T., Hengstler, JG., Kahl, R., Kramer, PJ., Schweinfurth, H. & Wollin, KM. (2008). Alternative methods to safety studies in experimental animals: role in the risk assessment of chemicals under the new European Chemicals Legislation (REACH). *Archives of Toxicology*, Vol. 82, No. 4, (April 2008), pp. 211-236, ISSN 1432-0738

Lindros, KO. (1997). Zonation of cytochrome P450 expression, drug metabolism and toxicity in liver. *General Pharmacology*, Vol. 28, No. 2, (February 1997), pp. 191-196, ISSN 0306-3623

Liu, H., Ye, Z., Kim, Y., Sharkis, S. & Jang, YY. (2010). Generation of endoderm-derived human induced pluripotent stem cells from primary hepatocytes. *Hepatology*, Vol. 51, No. 5, (May 2010), pp. 1810–1819, ISSN 1527-3350

Liu, H., Kim, Y., Sharkis, S., Marchionni, L. & Jang, YY. (2011). *In Vivo* Liver Regeneration Potential of Human Induced Pluripotent Stem Cells from Diverse Origins. *Science Translational Medicine*, Vol. 3, No. 82, (May 2011), p. 82ra39, ISSN 1946-6242

Liu, T., Zhang, S., Chen, X., Li, G. & Wang, Y.(2010). Hepatic differentiation of mouse embryonic stem cells in three-dimensional polymer scaffolds. *Tissue Engineering: Part A*, Vol. 16, No. 4, (April 2010), pp. 1115-1122, ISSN 1937-335X

Liu Tsang, V., Chen, AA., Cho, LM., Jadin, KD., Sah, RL., DeLong, S., West, JL. & Bhatia, SN. (2007). Fabrication of 3D hepatic tissues by additive photopatterning of cellular hydrogels. *The FASEB Journal*, Vol. 21, No. 3, (March 2007), pp.790–801, ISSN 1530-6860

Lu, C. & Li, AP. (2001). Species comparison in P450 induction: effects of dexamethasone, omeprazole, and rifampin on P450 isoforms 1A and 3A in primary cultured hepatocytes from man, Sprague-Dawley rat, minipig, and beagle dog. *Chemico-biological interactions*, Vol. 134, No. 3, (May 2001), pp. 271-281, ISSN 1872-7786

Mae, T., Inaba, T., Konishi, E., Hosoe, K. & Hidaka, T. (2000). Identification of enzymes responsible for rifalazil metabolism in human liver microsomes. *Xenobiotica*, Vol. 30, No. 6, (June 2000), pp. 565–574, ISSN 1366-5928

Maguire, T., Davidovich, AE., Wallenstein, EJ., Novik, E., Sharma, N., Pedersen, H., Androulakis, IP., Schloss, R. & Yarmush, M. (2007). Control of hepatic differentiation via cellular aggregation in an alginate microenvironment. *Biotechnology and Bioengineering*, Vol. 98, No. 3, (October 2007), pp. 631–644, ISSN 1097-0290

Malatesta, M., Perdoni, F., Santin, G., Battistelli, S., Muller, S. & Biggiogera, M. (2008). Hepatoma tissue culture (HTC) cells as a model for investigating the effects of low concentrations of herbicide on cell structure and function. *Toxicology in Vitro*, Vol. 22, No. 8, (December 2008), pp. 1853–1860, ISSN 1879-3177

Martin, Y. & Vermette, P. (2005). Bioreactors for tissue mass culture: design, characterization, and recent advances. *Biomaterials*, Vol. 26, No. 35, (December 2005), pp. 7481-7503, ISSN 1878-5905

Mazzoleni, G., Steimberg, N., Boniotti, J., Penza, L., Montani, C., Maggi, A., Ciana, P. & Di Lorenzo, D. (2008). Evaluation of Estrogen Receptor Interacting Compounds (ER-ICs) activity in a 3D ex-vivo model of mouse liver: comparison with the *in vivo* situation. *Proceedings of the Workshop "New animal models and in vitro systems for the pharmaco-toxicology of Nuclear Receptors Interacting Compounds (NR-ICs)"*, 24th European Congress of Comparative Endocrinology. Genova (Italy), (September 2008), pp. 23-24.

Mazzoleni, G., Di Lorenzo, D. & Steimberg, N. (2009). Modelling tissues in 3D: the next future of pharmaco-toxicology and food research? *Genes and Nutrition*, Vol. 4, No. 1 (March 2009), pp. 13-22, ISSN 1555-8932

Mazzoleni, G. & Steimberg, N. (2010). 3D culture in microgravity: a realistic alternative to experimental animal use. *Alternatives to Animal Experimentation*, Vol. 27, special issue, pp. 321-324, ISSN 0946-7785

Mazzoleni, G., Boukhechba, F., Steimberg, N., Boniotti, J., Bouler, JM. & Rochet, N. (2011). Impact of the dynamic culture condition in the RCCS™ bioreactor on a three-dimensional model of bone formation. *Procedia Engineering*, Vol. 10, pp. 3662-3667, ISSN 1877-7058

Meng, Q. (2010). Three-dimensional culture of hepatocytes for prediction of drug-induced hepatotoxicity. *Expert Opinion on Drug Metabolism and Toxicology*, (June 2010) Vol. 6, No. 6, pp. 733-746, ISSN 1742-5255

Meuwly, F., Ruffieux, PA., Kadouri, A. & von Stockar, U. (2007). Packed-bed bioreactors for mammalian cell culture: bioprocess and biomedical applications. *Biotechnology Advances*, Vol. 25, No. 1, (January-February 2007), pp. 45-56, ISSN 1873-1899

Miranda, JP., Rodrigues, A., Tostões, RM., Leite, S., Zimmerman, H., Carrondo, MJ. & Alves, PM. (2010). Extending hepatocyte functionality for drug-testing applications using high-viscosity alginate-encapsulated three-dimensional cultures in bioreactors. *Tissue Engineering, Part C*, Vol. 16, No. 6, (December 2010), pp. 1223-1232, ISSN 1937-3392

Mitzner, SR., Stange, J., Klammt, S., Peszynski, P., Schmidt, R. & Nöldge-Schomburg, G. (2001). Extracorporeal detoxification using the Molecular Adsorbent Recirculating System for critically ill patients with liver failure. *Journal of the American Society of Nephrology*, Vol. 12, No. suppl 17, (February 2001), pp. S75-S82, ISSN 1533-3450

Nahmias, Y., Berthiaume, F. & Yarmush, ML. (2006). Integration of technologies for hepatic tissue engineering. *Advances in Biochemical Engineering/Biotechnology*, Vol. 103, pp. 309-329, ISSN 1616-8542

Nakao, Y., Kimura, H., Sakai, Y. & Fujii, T. (2011). Bile canaliculi formation by aligning rat primary hepatocytes in a microfluidic device. *Biomicrofluidics*, Vol. 5, No. 2, (June 2011), pp. 22212-1-22212-7, ISSN 1932-1058

NRC Committee on Toxicity Testing and Assessment of Environmental Agents, National Research Council of the National Academies. Washington, D.C. (2007). *Toxicity Testing in the 21st century. A vision and a strategy.* Report of the Committee on Toxicity Testing and Assessment on Environmental Agents, The National Academies Press. Retrieved from http://www.nap.edu/catalog.php?record_id=11970

O'Brien, PJ., Irwin, W., Diaz, D., Howard-Cofield, E., Krejsa, CM., Slaughter, MR., Gao, B., Kaludercic, N., Angeline, A., Bernardi, P., Brain, P. & Hougham, C. (2006). High concordance of drug-induced human hepatotoxicity with *in vitro* cytotoxicity measured in a novel cell- based model using high content screening. *Archives of Toxicology*, Vol. 80, No. 9, (September 2006), pp. 580-604, ISSN 1432-0738

O'Brien, PJ., Chan, K. & Silber, P. (2004). Human and animal hepatocytes *in vitro* with extrapolation *in vivo*. *Chemico-Biological Interactions*, Vol. 150, No. 1, (November 2004), pp. 97-114, ISSN 1872-7786

Ohashi, K., Yokoyama, T., Yamato, M., Kuge, H., Kanehiro, H., Tsutsumi, M., Amanuma, T., Iwata, H., Yang, J., Okano, T. & Nakajima Y. (2007). Engineering functional two- and three-dimensional liver systems *in vivo* using hepatic tissue sheets. *Nature Medicine*, Vol. 13, No. 7, (July 2007), pp. 880-885, ISSN 1546-170

Ohno M., Motojima, K., Okano, T. & Taniguchi, A. (2008). Up-Regulation of Drug-Metabolizing Enzyme Genes in Layered Co-Culture of a Human Liver Cell Line and Endothelial Cells. *Tissue Engineering: Part A*, Vol. 14, No. 11, (November 2008), pp. 1861-186, ISSN 1937-335X

Okura, H., Komoda, H., Saga, A., Kakuta-Yamamoto, A., Hamada, Y., Fumimoto, Y., Lee, CM., Ichinose, A., Sawa,Y. & Matsuyama, A. (2010). Properties of hepatocyte-like cell clusters from human adipose tissue-derived mesenchymal stem cells. *Tissue Engineering: Part C*, Vol. 16, No. 4, (August 2010), pp. 761-770, ISSN 1937-3392

Omiecinski, CJ., Vanden Heuvel, JP, Perdew, GH. & Peters, JM. (2011). Xenobiotic metabolism, disposition, and regulation by receptors: from biochemical phenomenon to predictors of major toxicities. *Toxicological Sciences*, Vol. 120, No. Suppl1, (March 2011), pp. S49-75, ISSN 1096-0929

Pampaloni, F., Reynaud, EG. & Stelzer, EH. (2007). The third dimension bridges the gap between cell culture and live tissue. *Nature Reviews. Molecular Cell Biology*, Vol. 8, No. 10, (October 2007), pp. 839-845, ISSN 1471-0080

Park, K., Williams, DP., Naisbitt, DJ., Kitteringham, NR. & Pirmohamed, M. (2005). Investigation of toxic metabolites during drug development. *Toxicology and Applied Pharmacology*, Vol. 207, No. 2 suppl, (September 2005), pp. 425-434, ISSN 1096-0333

Pauli-Magnus, C. & Meier, PJ. (2003). Pharmacogenetics of hepatocellular transporters. *Pharmacogenetics*, Vol. 13, No. 4, (April 2003), pp. 189-198, ISSN 0960-314X

Payen, L., Courtois, A., Vernhet, L., Guillouzo, A. & Fardel, O. (1999). The Multidrug Resistance-Associated Protein (Mrp) Is Over-Expressed And Functional In Rat Hepatoma Cells. *International Journal of Cancer*, Vol. 81, No. 3, (May 1999), pp. 479–485, ISSN 1097-0215

Petersen, BE., Bowen, WC., Patrene, KD., Mars, WM., Sullivan, AK., Murase, N., Boggs, SS., Greenberger, JS. & Goff, JP. (1999). Bone marrow as a potential source of hepatic oval cells. *Science*, Vol. 284, No. 5417, (May 1999), pp. 1168–1170, ISSN 1095-9203

Popovic, JR. & Kozak, LJ. (2000). National hospital discharge survey: annual summary, 1998. *Vital Health Statitistics*, Vol. 13, No. 148, (September 2000), pp. 1-194, ISSN 0083-2006.

Rambhatla, L., Chiu, CP., Kundu, P., Peng, Y. & Carpenter, MK. (2003). Generation of hepatocyte-like cells from human embryonic stem cells. *Cell Transplantation*, Vol. 12, No. 1, pp. 1–11, ISSN 1555-3892

Rangarajan, A., Hong, SJ., Gifford, A. & Weinberg, RA. Species- and cell type-specific requirements for cellular transformation. *Cancer Cell*, Vol. 6, No. 2, (August 2004), pp. 171-183, ISSN 1878-3686

Rawden, H.C., Carilie, D.J., Tindall, A., Hallifax, D., Galetin, A., Ito, K. & Houston, JB. (2005). Microsomal prediction on in vivo clearance and associated interindividual variability of six benzodiazepines in humans. *Xenobiotica*, Vol. 35, No. 6, pp. 603–625, (June 2005), ISSN 1366-5928

Riccalton-Banks, L., Liew, C., Bhandari, R., Fry, J. & Shakesheff, K. (2003). Long-term culture of functional liver tissue: three-dimensional coculture of primary hepatocytes and stellate cells. *Tissue Engineering*, Vol. 9, No. 3, (June 2003), pp. 401-410, ISSN 1557-8690

Richert, L., Liguori, M.J., Abadie, C., Heyd, B., Mantion, G., Halkic, N. & Waring, J.F. (2006). Gene expression in human hepatocytes in suspension after isolation is similar to the liver of origin, is not affected by hepatocyte cold storage and cryopreservation, but is strongly changed after hepatocyte plating. *Drug Metabolism and Disposition*, Vol. 34, No. 5, (May 2006), pp. 870–879, ISSN 1521-009

Ring, A., Gerlach, J., Peters, G., Pazin, BJ., Minervini, CF., Turner, ME., Thompson, RL., Triolo, F., Gridelli, B. & Miki, T. (2010). Hepatic maturation of human fetal hepatocytes in four-compartment three-dimensional perfusion culture. *Tissue Engineering, Part C*, Vol. 16, No. 5, (October 2010), pp. 835-845, ISSN 1937-3392

Ruhnke, M., Ungefroren, H., Nussler, A., Martin, F., Brulport, M., Schormann, W., Hengstler, JG., Klapper, W., Ulrichs, K., Hutchinson, JA., Soria, B., Parwaresch, RM., Heeckt, P., Kremer, B. & Fändrich, F. (2005). Differentiation of *In Vitro*-Modified Human Peripheral Blood Monocytes Into Hepatocyte-like and Pancreatic Islet–like Cells. *Gastroenterology*, Vol. 128, No. 7, (June 2005), pp. 1774–1786, ISSN 1528-0012

Russel, W.M.S. & Burch, R.L. (1959). *The Principles of Humane Experimental Technique*, Methuen & Co. Ldt., London: pagg. 169-154, ISBN 0900767782 and now retrievable on http://altweb.jhsph.edu/pubs/books/humane_exp/het-toc

Schoonen, WG., Westerink, WM. & Horbach, GJ. (2009). High- throughput screening for analysis of *in vitro* toxicity. *Experientia*, Vol. 99, pp. 401–452, ISSN 1023-294

Schumacher, K., Khong, YM., Chang, S., Ni, J., Sun, W. & Yu, H. (2007). Perfusion culture improves the maintenance of cultured liver tissue slices. *Tissue Engineering*, Vol. 13, No. 1, (January 2007), pp. 197-205, ISSN 1557-8690

Shvartsman I., Dvir T., Harel-Adar T. & Cohen S. (2009). Perfusion cell seeding and cultivation induce the assembly of thick and functional hepatocellular tissue-like constructs. *Tissue Engineering: Part A*, Vol. 14, No. 4, (April 2009), pp. 751-760, ISSN 1937-335X

Schwartz, R.E., Reyes, M., Koodie, L., Jiang, Y., Blackstad, M., Lund, T., Lenvik, T., Johnson, S., Hu, W.S. & Verfaillie, C.M. (2002). Multipotent adult progenitor cells from bone marrow differentiate into functional hepatocytes. *Journal of Clinical Investigation*, Vol. 109, No. 10, (May 2002), pp. 1291–1302, ISSN 1558-8238

Schwarz, RP., Goodwin, TJ. & Wolf, DA. (1992). Cell culture for three-dimensional modeling in rotating-wall vessels: an application of simulated microgravity. *Journal of Tissue Culture Methods*, Vol. 14, No. 2, pp. 51-57, ISSN 0271-8057

Selden, C., Khalil, M. & Hodgson, HJF. (1999). What keeps hepatocytes on the straight and narrow? Maintaining differentiated function in the liver. *Gut*, Vol. 44, No. 4, (April 1999), pp. 443-446, ISSN 1468-3288

Şahin, S. (2003). Perfused Liver Preparation and its Applications. *FABAD Journal of Pharmaceutical Sciences*, Vol. 28, pp. 39-49, ISSN 300-4182

Si-Tayeb, K., Noto, FK., Nagaoka, M., Li, J., Battle, MA., Duris, C., North, PE., Dalton, S. & Duncan, SA. (2010). Highly efficient generation of human hepatocyte-like cells from induced pluripotent stem cells. *Hepatology*, Vol. 51, No. 1, (January 2010), pp. 297–305, ISSN 1527-3350

Sivaraman, A., Leach, JK., Townsend, S., Iida, T., Hogan, BJ., Stolz, DB., Fry, R., Samson, LD., Tannenbaum, SR. & Griffith, LG. (2005). A microscale *in vitro* physiological model of the liver: predictive screens for drug metabolism and enzyme induction. *Current Drug Metabolism*, Vol. 6, No. 6, (December 2005), pp. 569-591, ISSN 1875-5453

Slany, A., Haudek, V. J., Zwickl, H., Gundacker, N. C., Grusch, M., Weiss, T. S., Seir, K., Rodgarkia-Dara, C., Hellerbrand, C. & Gerner, C. (2010). Cell characterization by proteome profiling applied to primary hepatocytes and hepatocyte cell lines Hep-G2 and Hep-3B. *Journal of Proteome Research*, Vol. 9, No. 1, (January 2010), pp. 6–21, ISSN 1535-3907

Snykers, S., De Kock, J., Vanhaecke, T. & Rogiers, V. (2007). Differentiation of neonatal rat epithelial cells from biliary origin into immature hepatic cells by sequential exposure to hepatogenic cytokines and growth factors reflecting liver development. *Toxicology in Vitro*, Vol. 21, No. 7, (October 2007), pp. 1325–1331, ISSN 1879-3177

Soars, MG., McGinnity, DF., Grime, K. & Riley, RJ. (2007). The pivotal role of hepatocytes in drug discovery. *Chemico-biological interactions*, Vol. 168, No. 1, (May 2007), pp. 2-15, ISSN 1872-7786

Soto-Gutiérrez A., Navarro-Alvarez, N., Zhao, D., Rivas-Carrillo, JD., Lebkowski, J., Tanaka, N., Fox, IJ. & Kobayashi, N. (2007). Differentiation of mouse embryonic stem cells to hepatocyte-like cells by co-culture with human liver nonparenchymal cell lines. *Nature Protocols*, Vol. 2, No. 2, pp. 347-356, ISSN 1754-2189

Stephens, ML., Barrow, C., Andersen, ME., Boekelheide, K., Carmichael, PL., Holsapple, MP. & Lafranconi, M. (2012). Accelerating the development of 21st-century toxicology: outcome of a human toxicology project consortium workshop. *Toxicological Sciences*, Vol. 125, No.2, (February 2012), pp. 327-334, ISSN 1096-0929

Steimberg, N., Zarattini, G., Morandini, E., Pazzaglia, UE. & Mazzoleni, G. (2009). 3D culture of articular cartilage explants: new perspectives for future possible clinical applications. *The Journal of Bone Joint Surgery, British volume, Proceedings*, Vol. 91-B(II), pp: 269, ISSN 0301-620

Steimberg, N., Boniotti, J. & Mazzoleni, G. (2010). 3D culture of primary chondrocytes, cartilage, and Bone/cartilage explants in simulated microgravity. In: *Methods in Bioengineering: Alternative Technologies to Animal Testing*, Maguire and Novak, pp. 205- 212, ISBN 978-1-60807-011-4, Boston, USA

Sullivan, G.J., Hay, DC., Park, IH., Fletcher, J., Hannoun, Z., Payne, CM., Dalgetty, D., Black, JR., Ross, JA., Samuel, K., Wang, G., Daley, GQ., Lee, JH., Church, GM., Forbes, SJ., Iredale, JP. & Wilmut, I. (2010). Generation of functional human hepatic endoderm from human induced pluripotent stem cells. *Hepatology*, Vol. 51, No. 1, (January 2010), pp. 329–335, ISSN 1527-3350

Suzuki, H., Inoue, T., Matsushita, T., Kobayashi, K., Horii, I., Hirabayashi, Y. & Inoue T. (2008). In vitro gene expression analysis of hepatotoxic drugs in rat primary hepatocytes. *Journal of Applied Toxicology*, Vol. 28, No. 2, (March 2008), pp. 227-236, ISSN 1099-1263

Takahashi, K., Tanabe, K., Ohnuki, M., Narita, M., Ichisaka, T., Tomoda, K. & Yamanaka, S. (2007). Induction of pluripotent stem cells from adult human fibroblasts by defined factors. *Cell*, Vol. 131, No. 5, (November 2007), pp. 861–872, ISSN 1097-4172

Török, E., Pollok, JM., Ma, PX., Vogel, C., Dandri, M., Petersen, J., Burda, MR., Kaufmann, PM., Kluth, D. & Rogiers, X. (2001). Hepatic tissue engineering on 3-dimensional biodegradable polymers within a pulsatile flow bioreactor. *Digestive Surgery*, Vol. 18, No. 3, pp. 196-203, ISSN 1421-9883

Tosh, D., Shen, C. N. & Slack, J. M. (2002). Differentiated properties of hepatocytes induced from pancreatic cells. *Hepatology*, Vol. 36, No. 3, (September 2002), pp. 534–543, ISSN 1527-3350

Turner, R., Lozoya, O., Wang, Y., Cardinale, V., Gaudio, E., Alpini, G., Mendel, G., Wauthier, E., Barbier, C., Alvaro, D. & Reid, LM. (2011). Human hepatic stem cell and maturational liver lineage biology. *Hepatology*, Vol. 53, No. 3, (March 2011), pp. 1035-1045, ISSN 1527-3350

Unsworth, BR. & Lelkes, PI. (1998). Growing tissues in microgravity. *Nature Medicine*, Vol. 4, No. 8, (August 1998), pp. 901-907, ISSN 1546-170

U.S. EPA. (2009). The U.S. Environmental Protection Agency's Strategic Plan for Evaluating the Toxicity of Chemicals. Washington, DC: In *U.S. Environmental Protection Agency*. (2009). Available from http://www.epa.gov/spc/toxicitytesting/index.htm.

Valerio, LG. Jr. (2009). *In silico* toxicology for the pharmaceutical sciences. *Toxicology and Applied Pharmacology*, Vol. 241, No. 3, (December 2009), pp. 356–370, ISSN 1096-0333

Van de Bovenkamp, M., Groothuis, GMM., Meijer, DKF. & Olinga, P. (2007). Liver fibrosis *in vitro*: cell culture models and precision-cut liver slices. *Toxicology in Vitro*, Vol. 21, No. 4, (June 2007), pp. 545-557, ISSN 1879-3177

Vanhaecke, T., Snykers, S., Rogiers, V., Garthoff, B., Castell, JV. & Hengstler, JG. (2009). EU research activities in alternative testing strategies: current status and future perspectives. *Archives of Toxicology*, Vol. 83, No. 12, (December 2009), pp.1037-1042, ISSN 1432-0738

Vickers, AE., Fisher, R., Olinga, P. & Dial, S. (2011). Repair pathways evident in human liver organ slices. *Toxicology in Vitro*, Vol. 25, No. 7, (October 2011), pp.1485-1492, ISSN 1879-3177

Vunjak-Novakovic, G., Searby, N., De Luis, J. & Freed, LE. (2002). Microgravity studies of cells and tissues. *Annals of the New York Academy of Sciences*, Vol. 974, pp. 504-517, ISSN 1749-6632

Walker, TM. & Woodrooffe, AJ. (2001) Cytochrome P450 activity in control and induced long-term cultures of rat hepatocyte spheroids. *Toxicology in Vitro*, Vol. 15, No. 6, (December 2001), pp. 713–719, ISSN 1879-3177

Wang, S., Nagrath, D., Chen, PC., Berthiaume, F. & Yarmush, ML. (2008). Three-dimensional primary hepatocyte culture in synthetic self-assembling peptide hydrogel. *Tissue Engineering: Part A*, Vol. 14, No. 2, (February 2008), pp. 1-10, ISSN 1937-335

Werner, A., Duvar, S., Müthing, J., Büntemeyer, H., Lüsdorf, H., Strauss, M. & Lehmann, J. (2000). Cultivation of Immortalized Human Hepatocytes HepZ on Macroporous CultiSpher G Microcarriers. *Biotechnology and Bioengineering*, Vol. 68, No. 1, (April 2000), pp. 59-70, ISSN 1097-0290

Whitebread, S., Hamon, J., Bojanic, D. & Urban L. (2005). *In vitro* safety pharmacology profiling: an essential tool for successful drug development. *Drug Discovery Today*, Vol. 10, No. 21, (November 2005), pp. 1421-1433, ISSN 1878-5832

Wilkening, S. & Bader, A. (2003). Influence of culture time on the expression of drug-metabolizing enzymes in primary human hepatocytes and hepatoma cell line HepG2. *Journal of Biochemical and Molecular Toxicology*, Vol. 17, No. 4, pp. 207–213, ISSN 1099-0461

Wurm, M., Lubei,V., Caronna, M., Hermann, M., Buttiglieri, S., Bodamer, O., Muehl A., Tetta C., Margreiter R. & Hengster P. (2009). Introduction of a novel prototype bioartificial liver support system utilizing small human hepatocytes in rotary culture. *Tissue Engineering Part A*, Vol. 15, No. 5, pp. 1063-1073, ISSN 1937-335X

Xu, JJ., Diaz, D. & O'Brien, PJ. (2004). Applications of cytotoxicity assays and pre-lethal mechanistic assays for assessment of human hepatotoxicity potential. *Chemico-Biological Interactions*, Vol. 150, No. 1, (November 2004), pp. 115-128, ISSN 1872-7786

Yoffe, B., Darlington, GJ., Soriano, HE., Krishnan, B., Risin, D., Pellis, NR. & Khaustov, VI. (1999). Cultures of human liver cells in simulated microgravity environment. *Advances in Space Research*, Vol. 24, No. 6, pp. 829-836, ISSN 0273-1177

Zhang, L., Theise, N., Chua, M. & Reid, LM. (2008). The Stem Cell Niche of Human Livers: Symmetry Between Development and Regeneration. *Hepatology*, Vol. 48, No. 5, (November 2008), pp. 1598-1607, ISSN 1527-3350

Zucco, F., De Angelis, I., Testai, E. & Stammati, A. (2004). Toxicology investigations with cell culture systems: 20 years after. *Toxicology in Vitro*, Vol. 18, No. 2, (April 2004), pp. 153-163, ISSN 1879-3177

Permissions

The contributors of this book come from diverse backgrounds, making this book a truly international effort. This book will bring forth new frontiers with its revolutionizing research information and detailed analysis of the nascent developments around the world.

We would like to thank Michael G. Tyshenko PhD, MPA, for lending his expertise to make the book truly unique. He has played a crucial role in the development of this book. Without his invaluable contribution this book wouldn't have been possible. He has made vital efforts to compile up to date information on the varied aspects of this subject to make this book a valuable addition to the collection of many professionals and students.

This book was conceptualized with the vision of imparting up-to-date information and advanced data in this field. To ensure the same, a matchless editorial board was set up. Every individual on the board went through rigorous rounds of assessment to prove their worth. After which they invested a large part of their time researching and compiling the most relevant data for our readers. Conferences and sessions were held from time to time between the editorial board and the contributing authors to present the data in the most comprehensible form. The editorial team has worked tirelessly to provide valuable and valid information to help people across the globe.

Every chapter published in this book has been scrutinized by our experts. Their significance has been extensively debated. The topics covered herein carry significant findings which will fuel the growth of the discipline. They may even be implemented as practical applications or may be referred to as a beginning point for another development. Chapters in this book were first published by InTech; hereby published with permission under the Creative Commons Attribution License or equivalent.

The editorial board has been involved in producing this book since its inception. They have spent rigorous hours researching and exploring the diverse topics which have resulted in the successful publishing of this book. They have passed on their knowledge of decades through this book. To expedite this challenging task, the publisher supported the team at every step. A small team of assistant editors was also appointed to further simplify the editing procedure and attain best results for the readers.

Our editorial team has been hand-picked from every corner of the world. Their multi-ethnicity adds dynamic inputs to the discussions which result in innovative outcomes. These outcomes are then further discussed with the researchers and contributors who give their valuable feedback and opinion regarding the same. The feedback is then collaborated with the researches and they are edited in a comprehensive manner to aid the understanding of the subject.

Apart from the editorial board, the designing team has also invested a significant amount of their time in understanding the subject and creating the most relevant covers. They scrutinized every image to scout for the most suitable representation of the subject and create an appropriate cover for the book.

The publishing team has been involved in this book since its early stages. They were actively engaged in every process, be it collecting the data, connecting with the contributors or procuring relevant information. The team has been an ardent support to the editorial, designing and production team. Their endless efforts to recruit the best for this project, has resulted in the accomplishment of this book. They are a veteran in the field of academics and their pool of knowledge is as vast as their experience in printing. Their expertise and guidance has proved useful at every step. Their uncompromising quality standards have made this book an exceptional effort. Their encouragement from time to time has been an inspiration for everyone.

The publisher and the editorial board hope that this book will prove to be a valuable piece of knowledge for researchers, students, practitioners and scholars across the globe.

List of Contributors

Maria Paola Rubinetto, Nicola Petti and Lorenzo Rubinetto
Se.M. s.r.l. Medical Services, Cuneo, Italy

Gian Luca Rosso
Occupational Health Physician, Occupational Health Physician, S.C. Emergenza Urgenza 118, Cuneo, Italy

Mauro Feola
Riabilitazione Cardiologica – Unità Scompenso Cardiaco, Ospedale SS Trinità Fossano (CN), Italy

Tamer Oraby, Mustafa Al-Zoughool and Michael G. Tyshenko
McLaughlin Centre for Population Health Risk Assessment, University of Ottawa, Canada

Susie Elsaadany, Robert Gervais and Jun Wu
Public Health Agency of Canada, Ottawa, Canada

Lynn Johnston
Queen Elizabeth II Health Sciences Centre, Nova Scotia, Canada

Mel Krajden
BC Centre for Disease Control, University of British Columbia, Vancouver, Canada

Dick Zoutman
Medical Microbiology and Infection Control, Queen's University, Ontario, Canada

Daniel Krewski
McLaughlin Center for Population Health Risk Assessment, University of Ottawa, Ottawa, Canada
Department of Epidemiology and Community Medicine, Faculty of Medicine, University of Ottawa, Ottawa, Canada

Jinxiang Xi
University of Arkansas at Little Rock, Little Rock, AR, USA
Central Michigan University, Mount Pleasant, MI, USA

JongWon Kim
University of Arkansas at Little Rock, Little Rock, AR, USA

Xiuhua A. Si
Calvin College, Grand Rapids, MI, USA

Giuseppe Barbiero
Interdisciplinary Research Institute on Sustainability, Italy
Università della Valle d'Aosta, Italy

Alice Benessia
Interdisciplinary Research Institute on Sustainability, Italy
Università degli studi di Torino, Italy

Michael G. Tyshenko and Tamer Oraby
McLaughlin Centre for Population Health Risk Assessment, Institute of Population Health, University of Ottawa, Ontario, Canada

Susie ElSaadany, Marian Laderoute and Jun Wu
Blood Safety Surveillance and Health Care Acquired Infections Division, Centre for Communicable Diseases and Infection Control, Public Health Agency of Canada, Ottawa, Ontario, Canada

Willy Aspinall
Aspinall and Associates, Cleveland House, High Street, and Earth Sciences, Bristol University, Bristol, United Kingdom

Daniel Krewski
McLaughlin Centre for Population Health Risk Assessment, Institute of Population Health, University of Ottawa, Ontario, Canada
Department of Epidemiology and Community Medicine, Faculty of Medicine, University of Ottawa, Ottawa, Ontario, Canada

Peter R. Ganz
Health Canada, Director's Office, Ottawa, Ontario, Canada

Chao Chen, Maria Spassova and Leonid Kopylev
National Center for Environmental Assessment, Office of Research and Development, Environmental Protection Agency, USA

Viacheslav Ageev, Boric Fomin, Oleg Fomin and Tamara Kachanova
Faculty of Innovations, Saint-Petersburg State Polytechnic University, Russia

Xi Zhao and Anne-Lise Børresen-Dale
Department of Genetics, Institute for Cancer Research, Oslo University Hospital, The Norwegian Radium Hospital, Montebello, Norway
Institute of Clinical Medicine, University of Oslo, Norway

Ole Christian Lingjærde
Biomedical Research Group, Department of Informatics, Faculty of Mathematics and Natural Sciences, University of Oslo, Norway
Center for Cancer Biomedicine, University of Oslo, Norway

Giovanna Mazzoleni and Nathalie Steimberg
Laboratory of Tissue Engineering, General Pathology & Immunology Unit, Faculty of Medicine and Surgery, University of Brescia, Italy

Printed in the USA
CPSIA information can be obtained
at www.ICGtesting.com
JSHW011401221024
72173JS00003B/384